Rooted

GLOBAL HERBAL WISDOM FOR
PREGNANCY & POSTPARTUM:

USAGE AND CAUTION

by
Lyani Powers

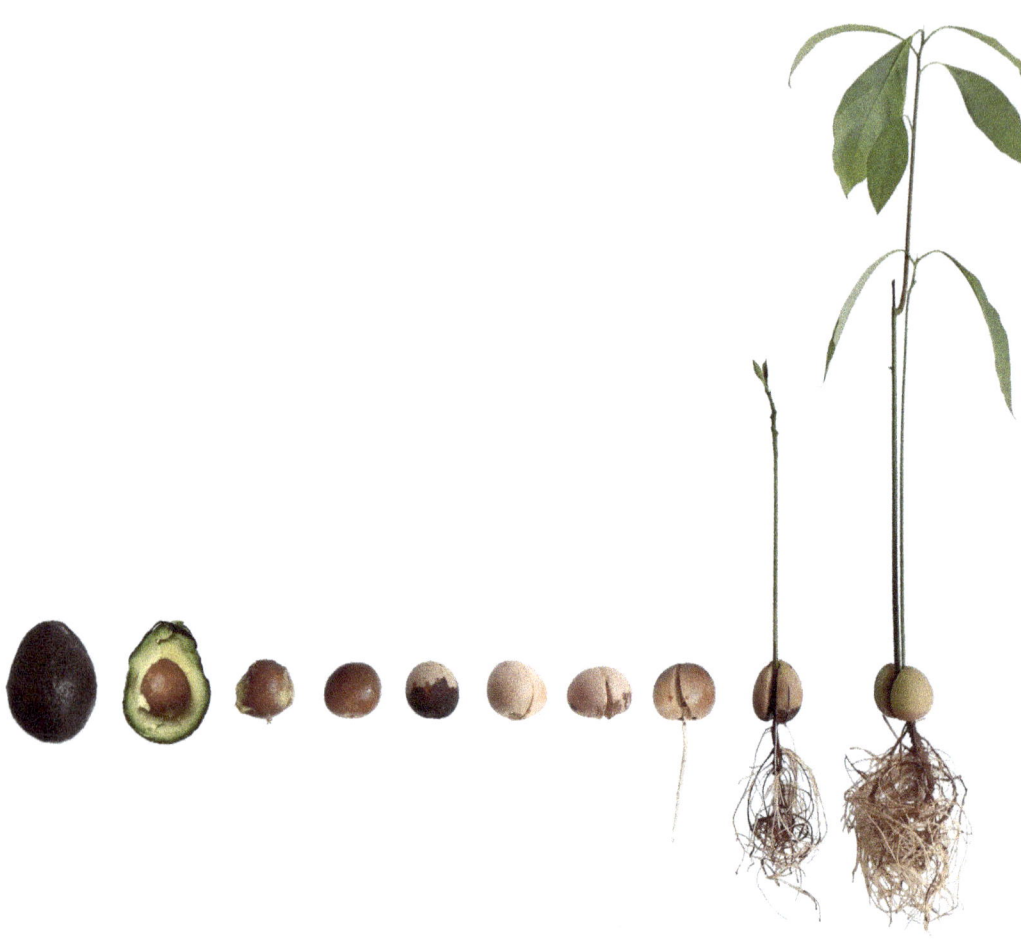

Disclaimer: The information provided in this book is for educational purposes only and is not intended as a substitute for professional medical advice, diagnosis, or treatment. This book does not replace the advice of a medical professional. Consult your physician before making any changes to your diet or regular health plan.

Copyright © 2024 Lyani Powers
All rights reserved.

ISBN#979-8-9919741-0-3

No part of this book may be reproduced or used in any manner without the prior written permission of the copyright owner, except for the use of brief quotations in a book review.

For my children, who are my
greatest teachers.
Love you more than french
fries and cupcakes...

--Mama

"In some Native Languages the term for plants translates to those who take care of us."

--Robin Wall Kimmerer
Author and Ethnobotanist

Table of Contents

Chapter 1:

Where Spirit and Science Meet p.8

Chapter 2:

Herbal Preparations and Herbal Actions p.34

Chapter 3:

Herbs to Avoid During Pregnancy p.48

Chapter 4:

Botanical Support For Pregnancy p.60

Chapter 5:

Herbs for Labor Support p.85

Chapter 6:

Botanical Support for Postpartum p.98

Chapter 7:

Breastfeeding and Galactogogues p.117

Chapter 8:

Ritual (Baths, Binding, Steams, & Ceremony) p.130

Chapter 9:

Nourishment p.170

Chapter 10:

Safety Guide and Resources & Index p.182

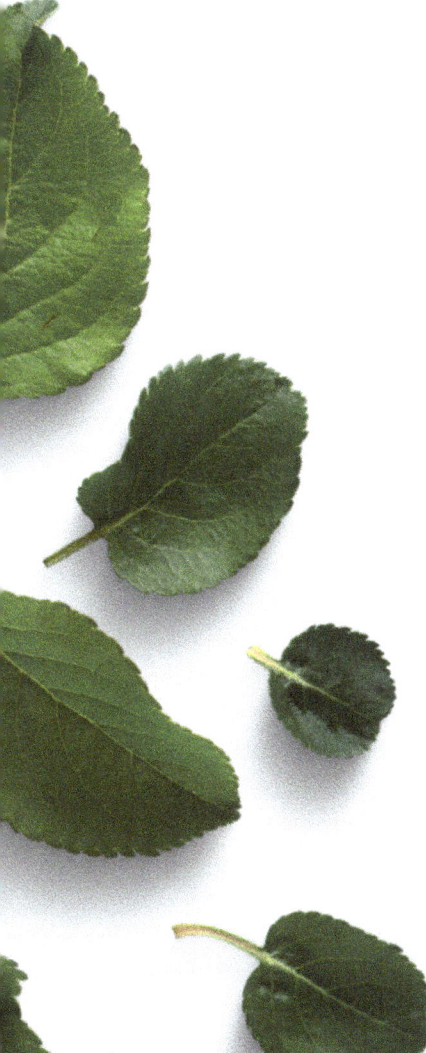

I created this guide to empower birthing individuals who often feel overwhelmed and helpless, turning to internet searches that leave them confused, anxious, and uncertain about how to use plants for support. Many resort to powering through discomfort or relying on over-the-counter solutions. The purpose of this project is to highlight natural alternatives and reintroduce birthing individuals to the plant allies that have supported this transformative and beautiful journey throughout history.

-Lyani Powers
xoxo

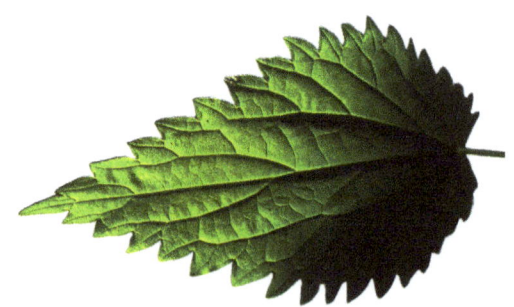

chapter 1

Dedication
Where Spirit and Science Meet
Holistic Approach
The Bias of "Research Based"
The Timeless Role of Herbs

"We began in her shade—running at her calloused heel, strapped to her strong back: the first mother, the one woman we all hold in common. Out of that band of 1,000 ancestors from whom humanity came, we rose like a dust storm out of the heart of Africa. But everyone in the menagerie came from the same litter, suckled at the same brown breast. And then, every one of her daughters changed through the generations. A tiny fragment of her flesh persists—a grain of earth she gave us."

Aurora Levins Morales

My Umi Said Share Your Light On the World

This book is dedicated to those who caught the babies—the women who answered the call and stood at the portal of life and death, often witnessing both sides of that door. In the dim light of a humble home, under the sheltering branches of an ancient tree, or within the sacred spaces of birth, birthworkers like Southern Black midwives such as Margaret Charles Smith, Indigenous midwives (parteras) like Martha Arotingo, my great-grandmother Francisca, a midwife in Cidra, Puerto Rico, and countless others like the Bean Feasas and Māori birthkeepers, have been steadfast guardians of life for generations. This book honors their legacy and the countless women around the world who have been pillars of their communities, preserving traditions that have sustained humanity for centuries.

These women, revered as wise elders and spiritual guides, carry the knowledge of birth in their hands and hearts, ensuring the safety and health of mothers, babies, and therefore all in their communities. They understood the deep connection between body, spirit, and community, offering care that extended beyond the physical act of childbirth. For them, birth was a sacred event requiring reverence, respect, and the tender touch of someone who understood the mysteries of life and death.

However, with the industrialization of birth in the 20th century, these midwives were increasingly marginalized. The rise of hospitals and the medicalization of childbirth often pushed them to the fringes as their practices were deemed outdated by a medical system that prioritized interventions and technology over tradition and intuition.

The conversation around modern birth practices is complex. While the modernization of birth has brought positive impacts, saving many lives through necessary interventions, it has also led to the unnecessary loss of traditional practices. This shift has had profound consequences, not just for mothers but for the healthcare system as a whole. When birth is treated solely as a medical event, divorced from its cultural and spiritual dimensions, it results in a disconnection that can harm both mothers and babies. This disconnection from the holistic, community-centered approach championed by these midwives has deprived both mothers and the healthcare system of the deep, empathetic care they provided.

The skills of Indigenous parteras have often been commodified and repackaged in private birthing centers where their ancient wisdom is sold as a luxury service rather than being recognized as a vital part of cultural heritage. While these centers offer a more personalized and holistic approach than traditional hospitals, they are often accessible only to those who can afford them, leaving many marginalized communities without the care they need. This privatization raises important questions about who benefits from this knowledge and who is left behind, emphasizing the need for these practices to be upheld and made accessible to all.

In Māori communities, the role of the *kuia* (elder women) and other birthkeepers has been integral in upholding the spiritual and cultural significance of birth. These birthkeepers, much like their counterparts in other Indigenous communities, embody a deep connection to the land, the ancestors, and the sacredness of life itself. Their practices are intertwined with tikanga (cultural practices) and whakapapa (genealogy), ensuring that each birth is honored as a continuation of the lineage and the spiritual connection between past, present, and future generations. They serve not only as midwives but as spiritual guides, cultural guardians, and protectors of the Māori way of life.

Today, in the face of dramatically high maternal mortality rates for Black mothers, there has been a powerful resurgence of Black birthworkers—midwives, doulas, and other advocates—who are reclaiming the traditions of their ancestors. These modern-day birthworkers are not just reviving old practices; they are revolutionizing the way we think about birth in the Black community. They are fighting against a system that has long ignored or mistreated Black mothers, offering an alternative rooted in empowerment, respect, and holistic care. These birthworkers are more than just practitioners; they are warriors in the fight for maternal justice, understanding the power of birth not only as a biological process but as a profound moment of empowerment for women.

High maternal mortality rates, particularly among Black mothers, and an increase in postpartum mood disorders highlight the critical need to return to a more holistic, community-centered approach to care—one that values the wisdom of traditional birthworkers and collaborates with them in caring for mothers and their families.

The resurgence of Black birthworkers is a powerful movement that benefits everyone. These modern-day birthworkers are revolutionizing the conversation around birth in the Black community, offering an alternative rooted in empowerment, respect, and holistic care. They are more than just practitioners; they are warriors in the fight for maternal justice, understanding the power of birth not only as a biological process but as a profound moment of empowerment for women.

The healthcare system itself stands to benefit immensely from honoring and incorporating the wisdom of traditional midwives. When traditional birth practices are upheld and respected, the system can better address the cultural, emotional, and spiritual needs of mothers, leading to better health outcomes and more positive birth experiences. Moreover, collaborative care that includes traditional midwives can reduce the strain on hospitals, lower the incidence of unnecessary interventions, and support a more sustainable, community-focused approach to maternal health.

By upholding and honoring the ways of these midwives, mothers benefit by preserving their right to compassionate, culturally resonant care, but we also strengthen the healthcare system as a whole, ensuring it remains rooted in the principles of holistic, community-centered support. Their work is a testament to the strength, resilience, and wisdom of women everywhere.

Looking to the future, one must continue to support and uplift the work of community birthworkers who carry on this legacy and remind us of the true power of birth and the importance of honoring it as the sacred act that it is. Let us never forget the contributions of these incredible women, and let us continue to fight for a world where every mother has access to the care, respect, and empowerment she deserves. In doing so, one not only honor the mothers who bring life into the world but also strengthen the healthcare system, ensuring that it serves all people with the compassion, wisdom, and reverence that birth deserves.

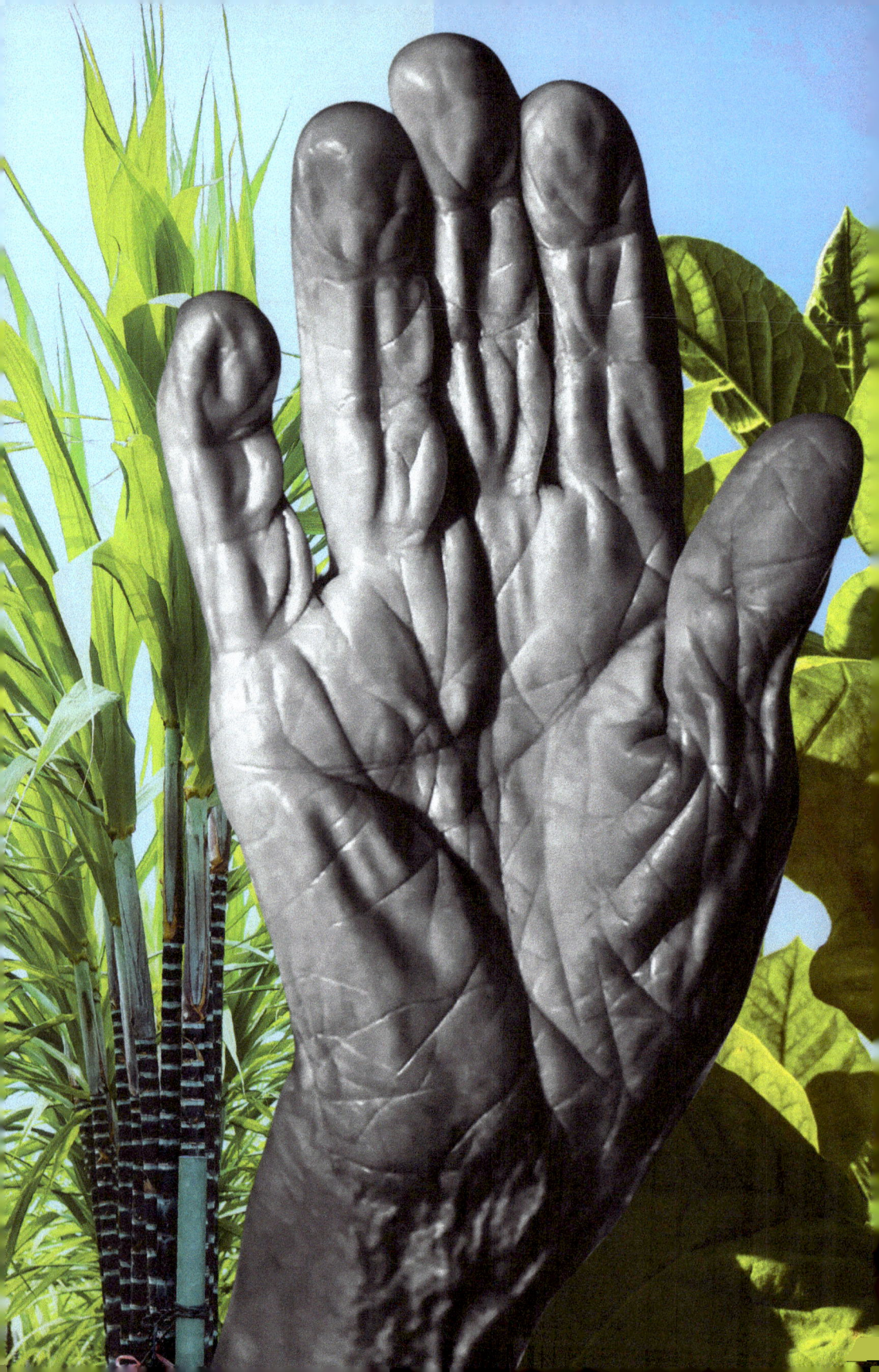

Remember Your Roots

Grandmothers are the spiritual anchors of the community and home. They are the keepers of sacred traditions, rituals, and stories passed down through generations, embodying the collective memory and spiritual resilience of their people. Their wisdom is not only practical but deeply connected to the land, the ancestors, and the spiritual well-being of the entire community. In many traditions, grandmothers play a crucial role in ceremonies, offering prayers, guidance, and blessings that nurture the spiritual growth of younger generations. Their presence is seen as a living bridge between the physical and spiritual realms, ensuring that the teachings of the ancestors are honored and carried forward with respect and love. They embody both the wisdom of lived experience and the nurturing spirit of ancestral continuity. From an anthropomorphic perspective, their role mirrors the behaviors observed in elephants and whales, who, like our elders, often live long past their reproductive years. These majestic animals use their extended lifespans to impart crucial survival knowledge and support the younger generations, ensuring the continuation of their lineage. Elephants, for instance, are known for their matriarchal societies, where the oldest females guide the herd with their profound knowledge of migration routes and resource locations. Similarly, whales, particularly orcas, benefit from the matriarchal leadership, where older females share their expertise on hunting and social behaviors. Spiritually, grandmothers represent the embodiment of ancestral wisdom, serving as conduits between past and future generations. Their presence is a sacred link to traditions, offering guidance, comfort, and a deep sense of belonging. By integrating their wisdom into community life, they help weave a rich tapestry of cultural identity and continuity, enriching the lives of younger members with both practical knowledge and spiritual depth.

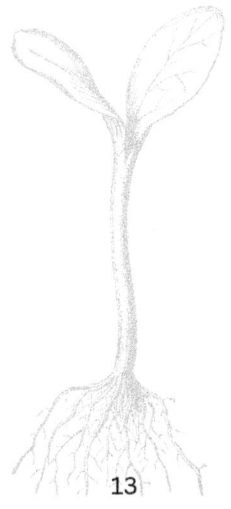

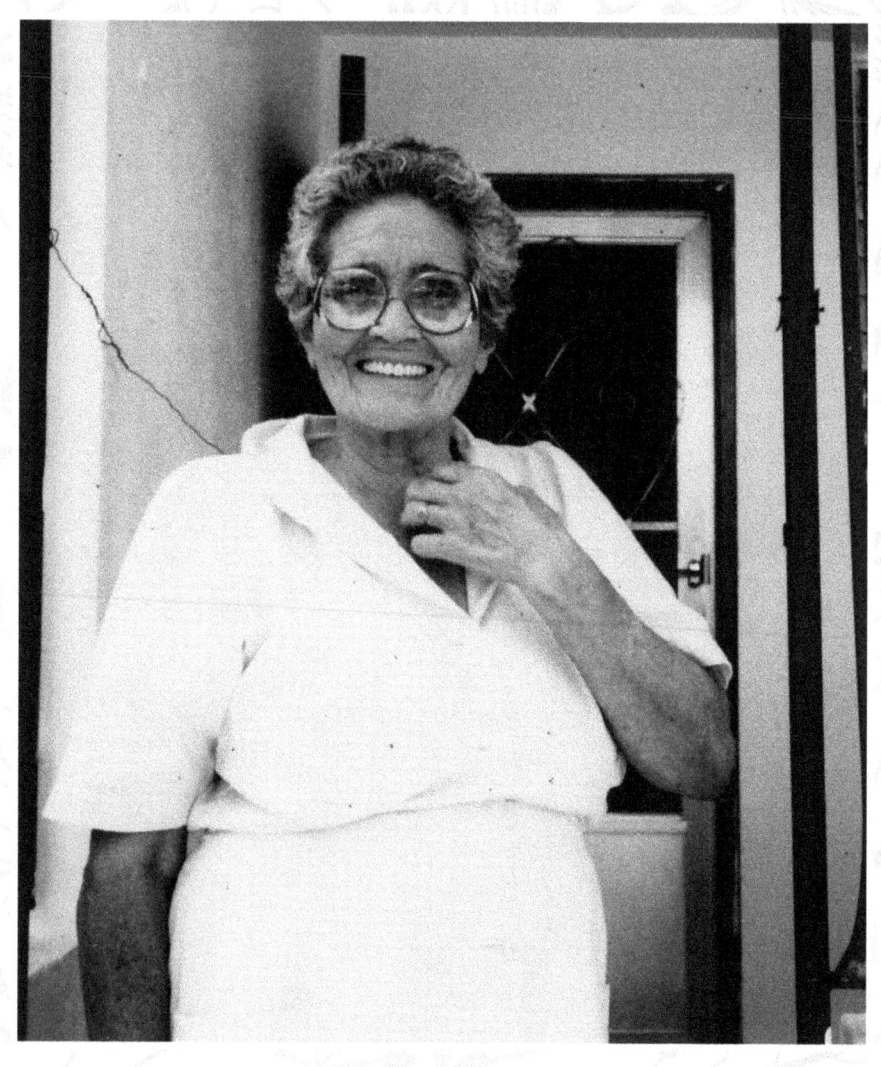

Francisca Reyes
Midwife, Mother of 11, My Great Grandmother

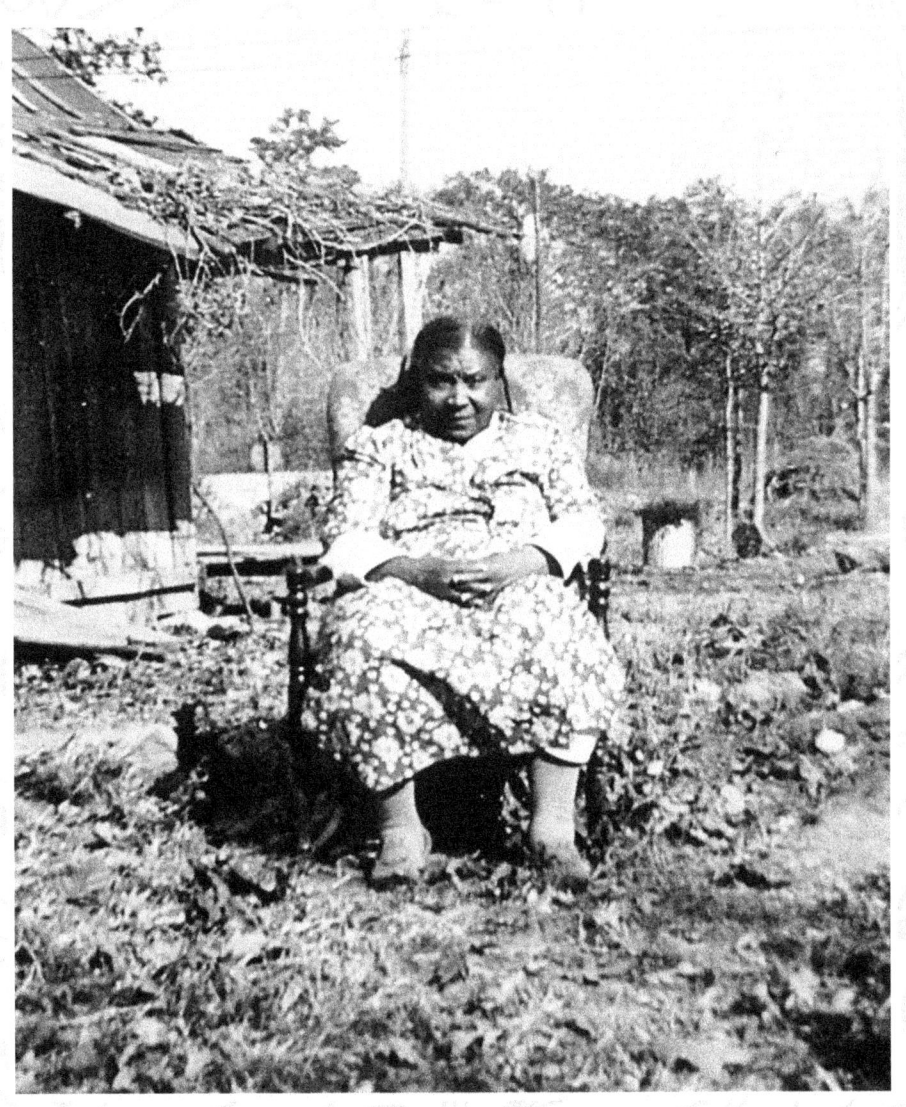

Maggie Clark

Farmer, Mother of 9, My Great Grandmother

"The land is always there. It is you who has to return to it."

Yusef Komunyakaa, Poet

Rooted Reflection

Take a deep breath in, and as you exhale, feel yourself becoming fully present in this moment. Close your eyes, and let your mind settle. Allow your body to relax, letting go of any tension with each breath.

Now, imagine yourself standing in a beautiful, sacred space—a place where you feel safe, connected, and grounded. This space is filled with warmth and light, and as you stand here, you become aware of the presence of countless women surrounding you.
These are the grandmothers of your lineage, the women who lived before you, each one a thread in the tapestry of your existence. As you breathe in, feel their energy, their wisdom, their strength flowing into you.

Visualize a long line of women stretching back through time. You are the culmination of their journeys, their love, their resilience. From the very first grandmother, who walked the earth thousands of years ago, to your own mother, each has played a role in bringing you here today.

There are 8,000 grandmothers in this lineage, each one a vital link in the chain of life that leads to you. With every breath, honor them. Feel their presence, their stories, their sacrifices. They are with you, always, supporting you, guiding you.

Now, place your hands over your heart, and silently thank these grandmothers. Thank them for the life they gave, for the wisdom they passed down, for the love that continues to flow through you. You are their legacy, their living prayer.

As you continue to breathe deeply, imagine sending your gratitude back through the line, reaching every grandmother in your lineage. See this gratitude as a golden light, flowing from your heart to theirs, connecting you across time and space.

Know that you are never alone. You carry the strength and spirit of 8,000 grandmothers within you. Whenever you need guidance or comfort, you can call upon them. They are a part of you, and you are a part of them.

Take one more deep breath, and as you exhale, feel the deep connection you share with these women. When you are ready, gently open your eyes, bringing this sense of connection and gratitude with you into your day.

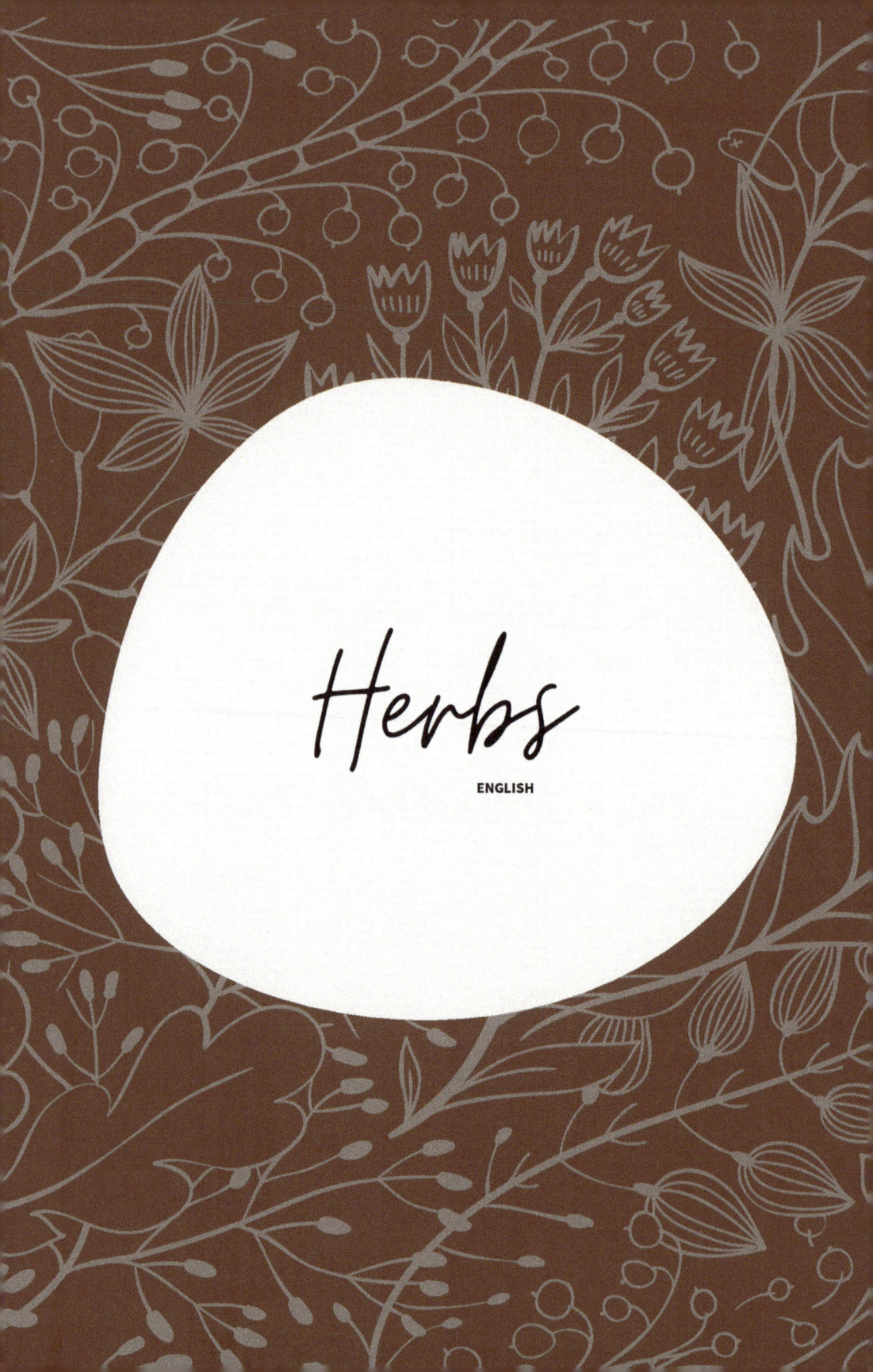

Herbs

ENGLISH

Where Spirit and Science Meet

My first teachers were my family. I often say I learned at the bottom of my grandmothers' skirts, absorbing their wisdom of plants and healing. My father also taught me about tending to the soul. His caramel hands, covered in freshly turned dirt, proudly held up a zucchini the length of his forearm or popped a sun-warmed tomato into my mouth. His skin matched the sunbaked earth beneath him, and like his mother, Barbara Clark, he could grow anything. I remember her, hinged at the hip with a hoe in hand, surrounded by greens up to her knees. Her hair wrapped, skin immaculate and ageless, she was a figure of beauty and wisdom. Her eleven children called her Mama, and her grandbabies, myself included, called her Nanny. She taught me many things, and I am grateful for them all.

My other grandmother, Petra, also shared her plant wisdom with me. Her garden was full of avocado, noni, mamajuana, thyme, plantain, cassava, rue, and so much more. Each visit was a lesson as she walked among the plants, touching each one and telling me its power, how to use it, and how to grow it. From my short height, she was the tallest tree in that garden. She is still in my life as I write this, and at 93, when I visit, she still takes me out to the garden to see what is growing. Although I now tower over her, she is still larger than life to me.

However, as I grew older and began speaking with other herbalists and botanists, and started to surround myself with people in academia, I began to feel that what I learned from my family was insufficient. The plant names I knew felt like family names, not the foreign scientific ones. I set about learning and mastering this new language, enrolling in ethnobotanical and clinical herbalism courses, and completing certification after certification. Yet, after all that, I felt like something was still missing. Upon reflection, I realized that all I had learned was incomplete without the original passion, the spirit of the plants, and the relationship with them—something I could never learn from a book.

So, I returned to the beginning to find the balance between spirit and science. I embraced the memories of my great and grandmothers and found all I needed in that connection. Now, I am back in communion with the plants. I speak to them in my first language or in Latin, or prayer if they prefer. The realization that both the scientific and the spiritual are needed has been transformative. It has brought me full circle and allowed me to honor my roots while integrating new perspectives, respecting and preserving traditional knowledge while also embracing modern insights.

Holistic Well-Being:
Integrating Mind, Community, Body, Ritual, and Spirit

In the pursuit of holistic well-being, it is essential to recognize the intricate interplay between the mind, community, body, ritual, and spirit. Each component plays a crucial role in fostering balance and promoting overall wellness. This integrative model emphasizes the importance of harmonizing various practices and perspectives, including the supportive use of herbs, nourishment, and conventional care.

Mind
The mind is central to our overall health. Our mental and emotional states deeply influence our physical health and our capacity to handle stress, make decisions, and interact with the world. Practices such as mindfulness, meditation, and cognitive-behavioral techniques are fundamental in nurturing mental well-being. They help manage stress, enhance focus, and cultivate a positive outlook, which in turn supports physical health and enriches our connection to our community and spirit.

Body
Our physical health reflects how well we care for our bodies. This involves not only addressing illness but also promoting overall wellness through regular exercise, balanced nutrition, and adequate rest. The body responds to both external and internal influences, such as stress and environmental factors. Practices like yoga, tai chi, and consistent physical activity are essential for maintaining bodily health and supporting natural healing processes.

Community
Community provides a vital support system that enriches our lives and fosters a sense of belonging. A strong, nurturing community offers emotional support, practical assistance, and shared wisdom. Engaging with community resources, participating in group activities, and building robust social networks are crucial for mental and physical health. Communities also contribute to the preservation and sharing of traditional practices, including herbal remedies and rituals that connect us to our cultural heritage.

Herbs & Nourishment
Herbs and nourishment are foundational elements of holistic health and integral to community wellness. Herbs have long been utilized to support various aspects of health, from digestive issues to emotional balance. Proper nutrition, including a diet rich in vitamins, minerals, and antioxidants, supports bodily functions and overall vitality. Integrating herbal remedies with conventional treatments can enhance their efficacy and provide additional support for maintaining health.

Ritual

Rituals and practices—whether cultural, spiritual, or personal—impart structure and meaning to our lives. They offer continuity and connect us to something larger than ourselves. Rituals can encompass daily routines, ceremonies, or traditional practices that mark significant life events, such as births, marriages, and seasonal changes. These practices enhance mental well-being, provide comfort, and deepen our connection to the spirit.

Spirit

The spirit represents our inner self, values, and connection to the greater whole. Spiritual practices, whether religious or secular, offer guidance, purpose, and a sense of inner peace. Engaging in spiritual practices may involve meditation, prayer, reflection, or simply spending time in nature. A strong spiritual connection enhances emotional resilience, fosters a sense of purpose, and supports overall well-being.

Midwives and Conventional Care

Midwives and doctors play essential roles in the healthcare landscape. Midwives offer specialized care in childbirth and postnatal support, often integrating traditional and holistic approaches. Doctors provide comprehensive medical care, including diagnosis, treatment, and management of health conditions. Medication, when necessary, addresses specific health issues and supports recovery. A collaborative approach between midwives, doctors, and patients ensures that all aspects of health—physical, emotional, and spiritual—are thoughtfully addressed.

Collaborative Approach

A holistic approach to health benefits from collaboration across various modalities. This includes the use of herbs and nourishment, which offer natural support for the body and mind, alongside conventional medical care. Working together with midwives, doctors, and other healthcare professionals ensures comprehensive care. Each practitioner contributes unique expertise and perspectives, creating a well-rounded framework for maintaining and enhancing health.

In summary, holistic well-being encompasses the mind, community, body, ritual, and spirit. Each element contributes to our overall health, and collaboration among diverse health practices and professionals—incorporating herbs, nourishment, and conventional medicine—creates a supportive and integrated approach to well-being.

"Plants and people coevolve. They become entangled in each other's lives. Our fate is inextricably linked with that of the plants that feed us, heal us, and give us shelter."

Gina Rae La Cerva
Anthropologist and Author

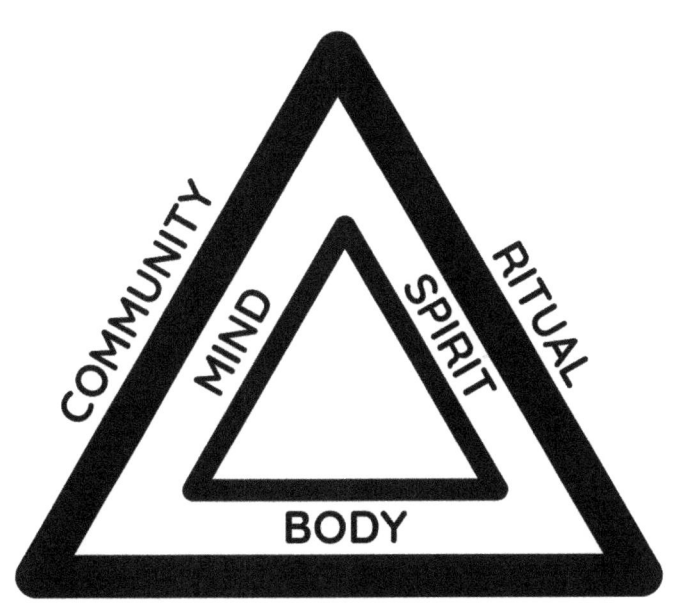

COLLABORATIVE HOLISTIC SUPPORT

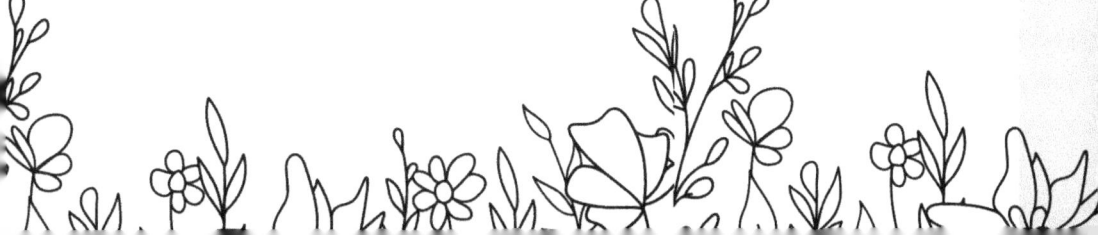

Decolonizing Herbalism: Integrating Folk Wisdom into "Research-Based" Standards

In the realm of herbalism, the term "research-based" often denotes a preference for scientific validation and clinical trials. While this approach has its merits in establishing safety and efficacy, it also reveals a significant injustice. This injustice arises from the underrepresentation and undervaluation of traditional knowledge systems, particularly those belonging to Indigenous, African, and other non-Western cultures. The dominance of Western scientific paradigms in herbalism has historically marginalized the rich and diverse herbal traditions of non-European cultures. For centuries, Indigenous peoples and communities of African descent have cultivated extensive knowledge of medicinal plants, passing down their uses through oral traditions and practical experience. However, these traditions often lack the formal documentation and standardized clinical trials that Western medicine demands, leading to their dismissal as "unproven" or "unscientific."

Research-based herbalism tends to prioritize studies conducted within Western scientific frameworks, which often do not account for the cultural and contextual nuances of traditional practices. For example, plants widely used in African or Indigenous healing traditions might not be studied or respected if they don't fit the Western clinical model. This exclusion not only diminishes the value of these practices but also deprives the broader community of potentially effective herbal remedies. Scientific research, while valuable, has limitations. It often focuses on isolating active compounds, which can strip away the holistic context in which plants are used in traditional medicine. This reductionist approach overlooks the synergistic effects of whole plants and the complex interactions between various herbs in traditional formulations. Moreover, funding and research priorities often favor plants that are profitable or familiar to Western markets, sidelining lesser-known herbs that may be central to non-Western medical systems. There is also an ethical dimension to consider. When Western researchers "discover" and commercialize herbal remedies long used by marginalized communities, they often fail to acknowledge or compensate the original knowledge holders. This can lead to cultural appropriation and exploitation, further entrenching racial inequalities. To create a more holistic and inclusive practice, herbalists can integrate both scientific research and traditional folk wisdom. This approach not only enriches the practitioner's understanding of herbal medicine but also respects and preserves the cultural heritage of diverse communities.

The first step for an herbalist is to acknowledge and value the rich heritage of traditional knowledge. This involves recognizing the expertise of Indigenous, African, and other non-Western herbal traditions. Herbalists can actively seek out this knowledge by studying ethnobotany, participating in cultural exchanges, and engaging with community elders or traditional healers. Understanding the historical and cultural context of herbal practices can provide deeper insights into the uses and effects of different plants.

While traditional knowledge offers a wealth of practical experience and holistic understanding, scientific research can provide a different layer of validation and clarity. An herbalist can cross-reference traditional uses of herbs with contemporary scientific studies. For instance, if a particular plant is known in folk medicine for its anti-inflammatory properties, an herbalist can look for scientific studies that investigate the plant's chemical compounds and their effects. This dual approach can confirm and sometimes even expand the known benefits of the herb.

Traditional herbal practices often use whole plants or complex mixtures, believing in the synergistic effects of their components. While scientific research frequently focuses on isolating specific active compounds, herbalists can respect this holistic approach by using whole plants or balanced formulations in their practice. When recommending an herb, they can consider both the scientifically studied active ingredients and the traditional knowledge of how the plant is used in combination with others. When using traditional knowledge, it is crucial for herbalists to approach it with respect and sensitivity. This means giving credit to the cultures and communities from which the knowledge originates and ensuring that any use of this knowledge is done ethically. Herbalists can advocate for fair trade practices, support sustainable harvesting, and participate in initiatives that protect the intellectual property rights of Indigenous and marginalized communities.

An integrated approach allows herbalists to provide more personalized care. Understanding the patient's cultural background and beliefs about medicine can help in creating a treatment plan that resonates with them. For example, if a client comes from a cultural background that values herbal tea rituals, an herbalist can incorporate such practices into their wellness plan, blending it with evidence-based recommendations. The fields of both traditional herbalism and scientific research are constantly evolving. Herbalists should commit to lifelong learning, staying updated on the latest research while also remaining open to learning from traditional healers and communities. Attending workshops, reading ethnobotanical literature, and participating in professional networks can help herbalists maintain a balanced and informed practice.

An integrated approach allows herbalists to provide more personalized care. Understanding the patient's cultural background and beliefs about medicine can help in creating a treatment plan that resonates with them. For example, if a client comes from a cultural background that values herbal tea rituals, an herbalist can incorporate such practices into their wellness plan, blending it with evidence-based recommendations. The fields of both traditional herbalism and scientific research are constantly evolving. Herbalists should commit to lifelong learning, staying updated on the latest research while also remaining open to learning from traditional healers and communities. Attending workshops, reading ethnobotanical literature, and participating in professional networks can help herbalists maintain a balanced and informed practice.

Herbalists can also act as bridges between traditional and scientific communities. By sharing insights from traditional practices with researchers and vice versa, they can help create a more inclusive and comprehensive body of knowledge. This can lead to more culturally sensitive research and a broader acceptance of diverse healing traditions. By integrating scientific research with folk wisdom, herbalists can honor the rich diversity of herbal traditions while ensuring the safety and efficacy of their practices. This balanced approach not only enriches their own understanding but also fosters a more inclusive and respectful field of herbal medicine. In doing so, herbalists can offer well-rounded, culturally sensitive care that honors the full spectrum of human knowledge and experience in healing.

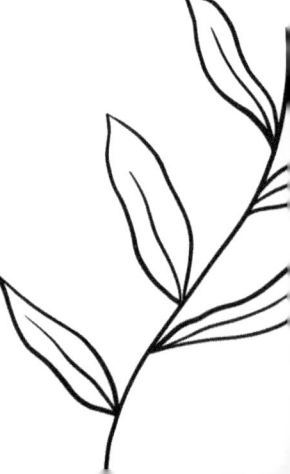

Ewe

YORUBA

Your Mama And Your Cousin Too

In my journey, I've come to see herbs as more than just plants—they're vital members of my community. This is in alignment with how most Indigenous cultures hold a profound respect for herbs, viewing them as relatives and even ancestors. In the context of community and family, especially when it comes to nurturing mothers and raising children, herbs play a crucial role. The adage "it takes a village to raise a child" encompasses not only human members of the community but also the natural environment, including herbs. These plant relatives contribute to the well-being of the community by providing medicinal support, nourishing foods, and spiritual guidance.

The practice of "mothering the mother" during pregnancy, childbirth, and postpartum involves a collective effort from the community to care for and support the mother, recognizing that a well-supported mother can better care for her child. Herbs are an essential part of this care, used to nourish, heal, and provide comfort. For example, herbal teas and baths are prepared to help soothe a mother's body and spirit, and specific plants are used to aid in recovery and promote milk production. This holistic approach to care acknowledges the physical, emotional, and spiritual needs of the mother. Elders and healers pass down knowledge about the uses of various plants, teaching younger generations to respect and understand the gifts of their plant relatives. This knowledge transfer is an essential part of cultural continuity and the community's collective wisdom.

In this way, herbs are not just passive elements in the environment but active participants in our community's life. They offer their healing properties willingly, and in return, they are honored and protected. They are not merely tools or resources, but essential partners in supporting the maternal dyad, offering their healing properties and wisdom. If we approach herbs in this perspective we can foster a deep sense of gratitude and responsibility towards the natural world. By honoring herbs as relatives, Indigenous cultures remind us of the importance of living in harmony with nature and respecting all forms of life. In doing so, they uphold a worldview that cherishes interdependence, community, and the sacredness of the bond between mother and child during pregnancy and postpartum.

Roots and Rituals: The Timeless Role of Herbs

Throughout history, humans have had a profound and intricate relationship with plants, particularly herbs. This connection is deeply rooted in the ethnobotanical view, which examines how different cultures have used and perceived plants over time. From ancient civilizations to contemporary societies, herbs have played a crucial role in healing, spiritual practices, culinary traditions, and daily life.

Ancient Civilizations and Early Uses
The use of herbs dates back thousands of years, with evidence found in ancient texts, artifacts, and oral traditions. In the Kingdom of Kush, located in present-day Sudan, herbs played a significant role in daily life and medicine. Kush's strategic position along trade routes facilitated the exchange of botanical knowledge and resources, further enriching their herbal practices. In neighboring Egypt, herbs such as garlic, coriander, and aloe vera were documented in medical papyri and used for both medicinal and ritualistic purposes. Similarly, the Chinese Materia Medica, one of the oldest pharmacological texts, lists hundreds of herbs used in Traditional Chinese Medicine (TCM) for their healing properties.

In the Indian subcontinent, the practice of Ayurveda, which means "the science of life," has utilized herbs for over 5,000 years. Ayurvedic texts like the Charaka Samhita and Sushruta Samhita detail the medicinal uses of herbs like turmeric, ginger, and neem, emphasizing the balance of body, mind, and spirit.

Indigenous Knowledge and Ethnobotany
Indigenous cultures across the globe have long held deep knowledge of the local flora. This ethnobotanical wisdom has been passed down through generations, often orally, and includes a vast understanding of the medicinal, nutritional, and spiritual properties of herbs. For instance, Native American tribes have used herbs like sage, sweetgrass, and tobacco in ceremonial practices and healing rituals. These plants are not only seen as sources of medicine but also as sacred beings with spiritual significance.

In the Amazon rainforest, Indigenous peoples have a rich tradition of using plants for various purposes. For example, certain plants are used in spiritual ceremonies to induce visions and connect with the spirit world. The extensive knowledge of these plants is a testament to the deep respect and understanding that Indigenous peoples have for their natural environment.

Herbs in Spiritual and Cultural Practices
Herbs have also been integral to spiritual and cultural practices worldwide. In ancient Greece and Rome, herbs like bay laurel and myrrh were used in religious ceremonies and as offerings to the gods. In medieval Europe, herbs were often associated with magic and superstition, with plants like mandrake and belladonna being used in potions and spells. In Christianity, herbs like hyssop are mentioned in the Bible and were burned as incense in churches, symbolizing purification and sanctification. Similarly, frankincense and myrrh, gifted to the infant Jesus, held significant spiritual meaning and were valued for their aromatic and medicinal properties.

The use of herbs in spiritual practices is not just historical but continues in many cultures today. For example, in Afro-Caribbean traditions such as Santería and Vodou, herbs are used in rituals to communicate with spirits, protect against evil, and promote healing. These practices highlight the symbolic and energetic properties attributed to herbs. This deep connection between herbs and spiritual practices reflects the universal belief in the healing and protective powers of nature. It also highlights the cultural importance of plants in connecting humans with the divine and the natural world. Through these practices, herbs have been more than just physical remedies; they have been symbols of faith, healing, and the continuity of life.

Herbs in Modern Medicine and Cuisine
In contemporary times, the use of herbs has evolved and expanded. While modern medicine has developed synthetic drugs, the use of herbal remedies persists, often as complementary or alternative therapies. The resurgence of interest in natural and holistic health has led to the popularity of herbal supplements, teas, and essential oils.

Herbs also play a significant role in global cuisine. Culinary herbs like basil, rosemary, and cilantro not only enhance flavors but also offer health benefits. The culinary use of herbs often intersects with their medicinal properties, as seen in traditional dishes designed to promote digestion or boost immunity.

The Future of Ethnobotany and Herbalism
As the world becomes more interconnected, there is a growing recognition of the importance of preserving traditional knowledge and biodiversity. Ethnobotany, as a field, continues to document and study the relationships between people and plants, offering valuable insights into sustainable living and cultural heritage.

In conclusion, the history of herbs is a rich tapestry of cultural, spiritual, and medicinal traditions. Herbs have been and continue to be an essential part of human life, bridging the past and present, and offering a deep connection to nature. Through the lens of ethnobotany, we can appreciate the profound wisdom and respect that different cultures have cultivated towards these remarkable plants.

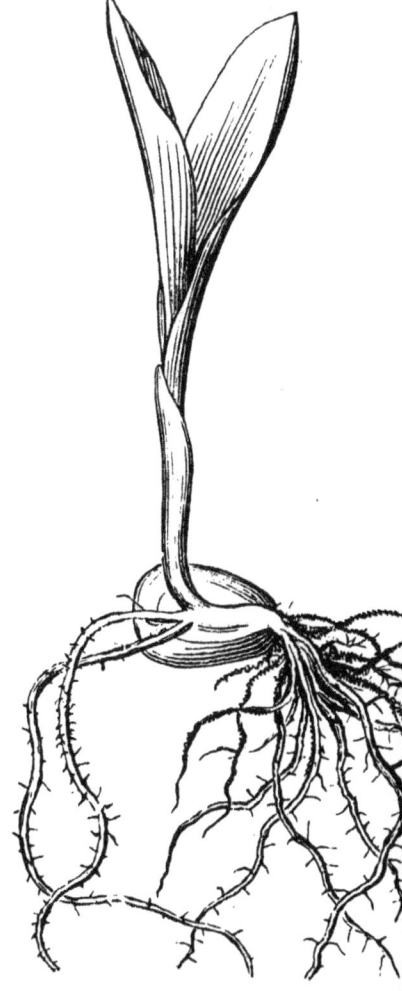

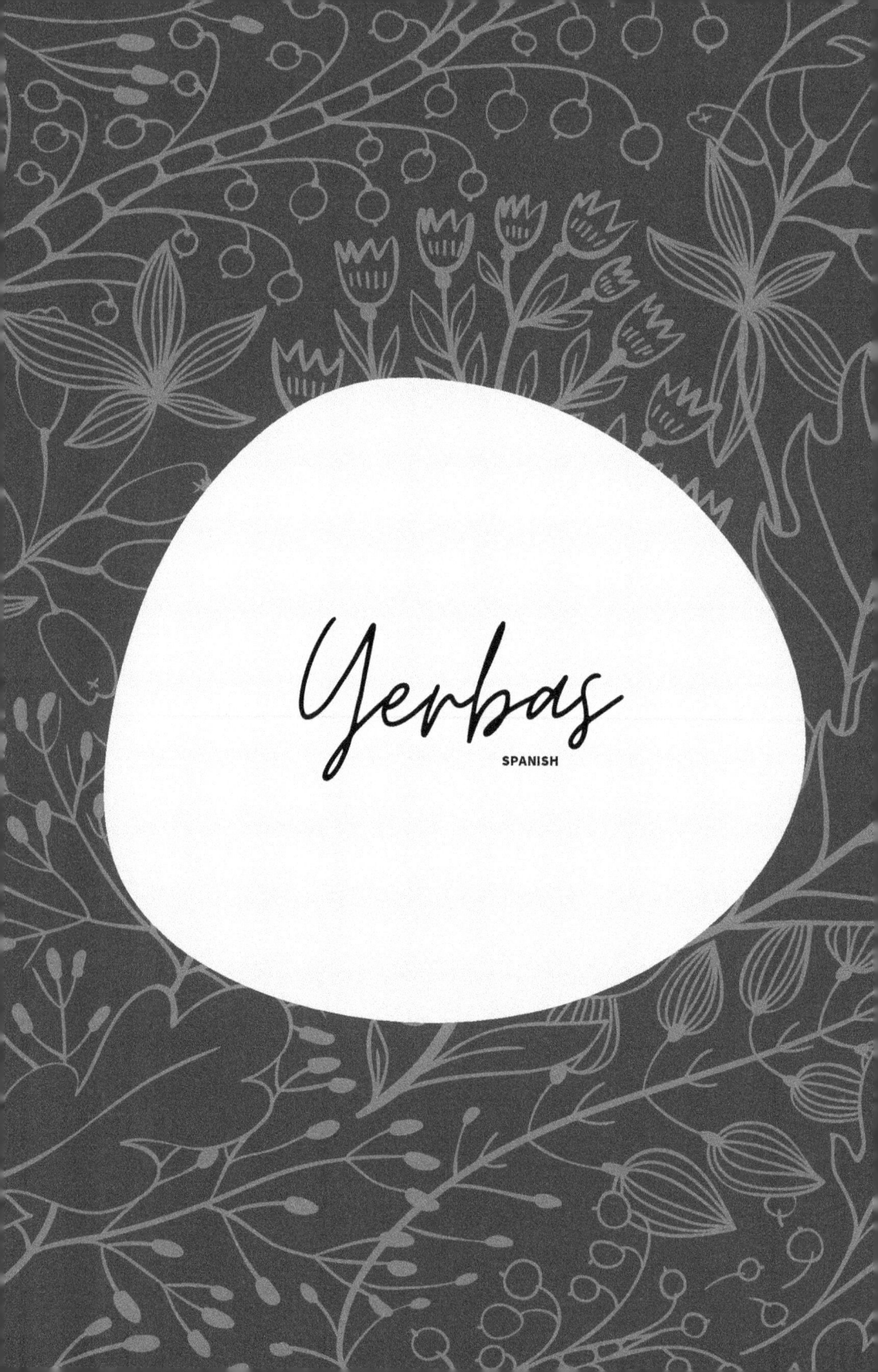
Yerbas
SPANISH

chapter 2

Guide To Herbal Preparations
Herbal Actions

A Guide to Herbal Preparations

Herbs have been used for centuries in various cultures for their medicinal, culinary, and spiritual properties. The ways in which herbs are prepared and administered can vary widely, depending on the desired effect and the specific plant's properties. Below is an overview of common herbal preparations and a list of herbal action categories, along with definitions and examples.

Teas (Infusions and Decoctions)
Infusions: Made by steeping delicate parts of herbs (like leaves and flowers) in hot water. This is similar to making a cup of tea. Infusions are typically used for more delicate herbs and are consumed hot or cold.
Decoctions: Involve simmering harder parts of herbs (such as roots, bark, or seeds) in water for a longer time to extract their active ingredients. Decoctions are generally more potent than infusions.

Poultice
A poultice is a soft, moist mass of herbs applied directly to the skin. The herbs are often crushed or chopped and mixed with a liquid (such as water or vinegar) to form a paste. Poultices are used to reduce inflammation, draw out toxins, or soothe irritated skin.

Compress
A compress involves soaking a cloth in an herbal infusion or decoction and then applying it to the skin. It can be hot or cold, depending on the desired effect. Compresses are often used for localized pain, swelling, or infections.

Tincture
Tinctures are concentrated herbal extracts made by soaking herbs in alcohol or a mixture of alcohol and water. They are typically more potent than teas and are taken in small doses, usually by the dropperful. Tinctures are convenient for long-term storage and use.

Syrup
Syrups are sweetened herbal preparations often used to make herbs more palatable, especially for children. They are made by combining an herbal decoction or infusion with a sweetener, like honey or sugar, and then reducing it to a thick consistency.

Elixir
Similar to tinctures but typically sweeter and sometimes containing glycerin or honey, elixirs combine the medicinal properties of herbs with the taste and soothing qualities of a sweetener. They are often used to treat coughs and soothe the throat.

Herbal teas can be prepared using different methods depending on the type of herb and desired effects. Here is a step-by-step guide to creating infusions, decoctions, and cold infusions, along with the types of herbs typically used for each method.

Infusions

Infusions are best for delicate parts of herbs, such as leaves, flowers, and some berries. This method extracts vitamins, volatile oils, and other beneficial compounds.

Common Herbs for Infusions:
- Leaves: Nettle, peppermint, raspberry leaf, lemon balm
- Flowers: Chamomile, hibiscus, elderflower, lavender
- Soft Berries: Hawthorn berries, rose hips

Instructions:
1. Measure the Herb: Use approximately 1 tablespoon of dried herbs (or 2 tablespoons of fresh herbs) per 8 ounces (1 cup) of water.
2. Boil Water: Bring water to a boil. Place the herbs in a teapot, mug, or heat-resistant jar. Pour the boiling water over the herbs.
3. Cover and Steep: Cover the container to keep the essential oils from escaping. Steep for 5-15 minutes, depending on the herb and desired strength.
4. Strain and Serve: Strain the herbs and pour the liquid into a cup. Sweeten with honey or another sweetener if desired.

Cold Infusions

Cold infusions are used for herbs whose beneficial properties may be degraded by heat. This method is also suitable for mucilaginous herbs.

Common Herbs for Cold Infusions:
- Mucilaginous Herbs: Marshmallow root, slippery elm bark, chia seeds
- Delicate Herbs: Mint, chamomile, rose petals

Instructions:
- Measure the Herb: Use approximately 1 tablespoon of dried herbs (or 2 tablespoons of fresh herbs) per 8 ounces (1 cup) of cold water.
- Add Cold Water: Place the herbs in a jar or pitcher and cover them with cold water.
- Cover and Refrigerate: Cover the container and let it sit in the refrigerator for 4-12 hours. The longer infusion time is often needed for mucilaginous herbs.
- Strain and Serve: Strain the herbs and serve the infusion cold. Sweeten if desired.

Decoctions

Decoctions are used for tougher plant materials such as roots, bark, seeds, and some berries. This method involves simmering the herbs to extract the beneficial compounds.

Common Herbs for Decoctions:
- Roots: Ginger, dandelion root, burdock root, licorice root
- Bark: Cinnamon bark, wild cherry bark
- Seeds: Fennel, cardamom, fenugreek
- Hard Berries: Juniper berries, schisandra berries

Instructions:
- Measure the Herb: Use approximately 1 tablespoon of dried herbs (or 2 tablespoons of fresh herbs) per 8 ounces (1 cup) of water.
- Combine Water and Herbs: Place the herbs and water in a saucepan.
- Boil and Simmer: Bring the water to a boil, then reduce the heat and let the herbs simmer for 20-45 minutes. The longer simmering time is often needed for harder plant materials.
- Strain and Serve: Strain the herbs and pour the liquid into a cup. Sweeten if desired.

Herbal Syrup

Herbal syrups are sweet, concentrated herbal extracts that can be taken by the spoonful or added to drinks. They are particularly useful for soothing the throat, boosting the immune system, or calming the stomach.

Common Herbs for Syrups:
- Immune Support: Elderberries, echinacea, rose hips
- Respiratory Health: Licorice root, ginger, thyme
- Digestive Health: Fennel, peppermint, ginger

Instructions:
1. Prepare the Herbal Decoction:
   - Measure 1 cup of dried herbs or 2 cups of fresh herbs per 1 quart (4 cups) of water. Alternatively, use approximately 1 tablespoon of dried herbs per 1 cup of water for smaller quantities.
   - Add herbs to water and bring to a boil, then reduce the heat and simmer for 15-30 minutes
2. Strain the Herbs:
   - Strain the liquid into a heat-resistant bowl or jar using a fine mesh strainer or cheesecloth. Squeeze out as much liquid as possible from the herbs.
3. Add Sweetener:
   - Measure the strained liquid and add an equal amount of sweetener (honey, sugar, or glycerin). For example, if you have 2 cups of herbal decoction, add 2 cups of sweetener.
   - If using honey, add it when the liquid has cooled slightly to preserve its beneficial properties.
4. Simmer and Thicken:
   - Return the mixture to the saucepan and gently simmer on low heat for an additional 10-15 minutes until it reaches a syrupy consistency. Stir occasionally.
5. Cool and Store:
   - Allow the syrup to cool, then pour it into sterilized glass jars or bottles. Store in the refrigerator for up to 3 months.

Herbal Poultice

A poultice is a soft, moist mass of herbs applied to the skin to relieve soreness, inflammation, or infection. It is a direct way to use herbs for topical treatment.

Common Herbs for Poultices:
- Inflammation and Pain Relief: Arnica, comfrey, calendula
- Infections and Abscesses: Garlic, onion, plantain
- Soothing Irritated Skin: Chamomile, marshmallow root, lavender

Instructions:
1. Prepare the Herbs:
    - Fresh Herbs: Crush or mash fresh herbs using a mortar and pestle or blender.
    - Dried Herbs: Mix dried herbs with warm water to create a paste.
2. Apply the Poultice:
    - Spread the herbal paste or mash onto a clean piece of cloth, gauze, or directly onto the skin.
    - Ensure the poultice covers the affected area completely.
3. Cover and Secure:
    - Cover the poultice with a second cloth or bandage to keep it in place. You can also wrap it with plastic wrap or a towel to retain warmth and moisture.
4. Leave in Place:
    - Leave the poultice on the skin for 20-30 minutes, or longer if comfortable and depending on the herbs used. Replace with a fresh poultice as needed.
5. Remove and Clean:
    - Gently remove the poultice and rinse the area with warm water. Repeat the application as necessary.

Guide to Making Herbal Tinctures

Tinctures are concentrated herbal extracts made by soaking herbs in alcohol or another solvent. They are a convenient way to consume herbal medicine, as they have a long shelf life and are easy to take.

Tincture with Fresh Herbs
Materials Needed:
- Fresh herbs
- Alcohol (80-100 proof vodka or brandy)
- Glass jar with a tight-fitting lid
- Cheesecloth or fine mesh strainer
- Dark glass dropper bottles for storage

Instructions:
1. Prepare the Fresh Herbs:
   - Rinse the fresh herbs to remove dirt and debris.
   - Chop the herbs finely to increase the surface area for extraction.
2. Fill the Jar:
   - Fill a clean glass jar about two-thirds full with the chopped fresh herbs.
3. Add Alcohol:
   - Pour alcohol over the herbs, covering them completely. Leave about an inch of space at the top of the jar. Ensure all herbs are submerged to prevent mold growth.
4. Seal and Store:
   - Seal the jar tightly and label it with the date and contents.
   - Store the jar in a cool, dark place for 4-6 weeks. Shake the jar gently every day or every few days to help the extraction process.
5. Strain the Tincture:
   - After 4-6 weeks, strain the mixture through cheesecloth or a fine mesh strainer into a clean bowl or jar. Squeeze out as much liquid as possible from the herbs.
6. Bottle and Store:
   - Pour the strained liquid into dark glass dropper bottles for storage. Label with the herb name and date. Store in a cool, dark place. Tinctures can last for several years.

Tincture with Dried Herbs

Materials Needed:
- Dried herbs
- Alcohol (80-100 proof vodka or brandy)
- Glass jar with a tight-fitting lid
- Cheesecloth or fine mesh strainer
- Dark glass dropper bottles for storage

Instructions:
- Prepare the Dried Herbs:
    - Measure the desired amount of dried herbs. Typically, use a ratio of 1 part dried herbs to 5 parts alcohol.
- Fill the Jar:
    - Place the dried herbs in a clean glass jar.
- Add Alcohol:
    - Pour alcohol over the dried herbs, ensuring they are fully submerged. Stir to remove air bubbles, and add more alcohol if needed.
- Seal and Store:
    - Seal the jar tightly and label it with the date and contents.
    - Store the jar in a cool, dark place for 4-6 weeks. Shake the jar gently every day or every few days to aid extraction.
- Strain the Tincture:
    - After 4-6 weeks, strain the mixture through cheesecloth or a fine mesh strainer into a clean bowl or jar. Press the herbs to extract as much liquid as possible.
- Bottle and Store:
    - Pour the strained liquid into dark glass dropper bottles for storage. Label with the herb name and date. Store in a cool, dark place. Tinctures can last for several years.

Additional Tips
- Choosing Alcohol: Use alcohol with a high enough proof (40-50% or 80-100 proof) to effectively extract the medicinal properties of the herbs and preserve the tincture.
- Safety: Always label your tinctures clearly with the contents and date made. Store out of reach of children.
- Dosage: Tinctures are potent; typically, only a few drops to a teaspoon are taken at a time. Consult a healthcare provider or herbalist for appropriate dosages.
- Non-Alcoholic Alternatives: For those who prefer to avoid alcohol, glycerin or vinegar can be used as a menstruum, though the extraction will be less potent and have a shorter shelf life.

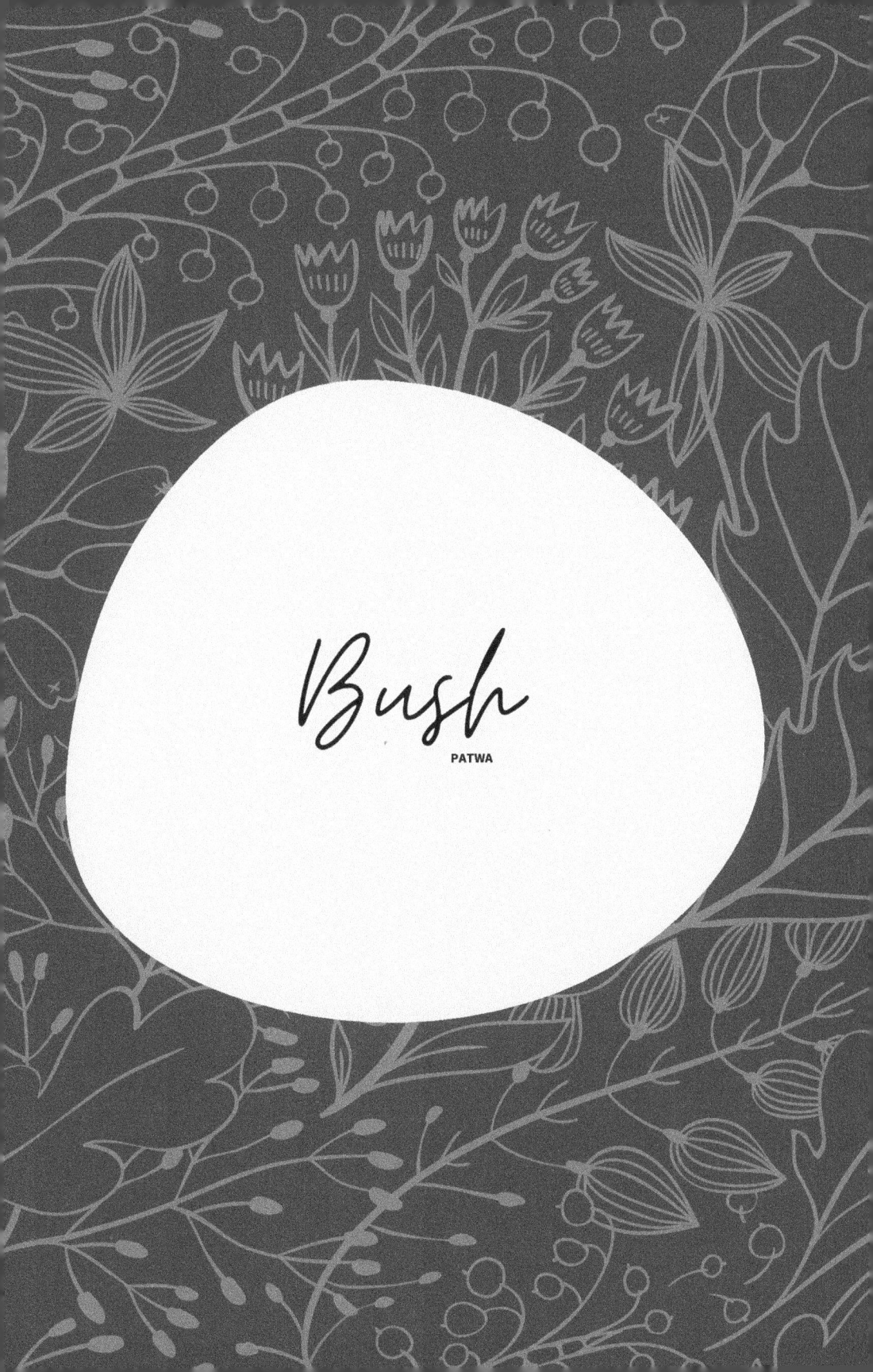

Bush

PATWA

Herbal Actions

Herbal actions describe the effects that herbs have on the body, helping to categorize them based on their therapeutic effects. This categorization guides their use in treating various conditions. Understanding these actions and preparations forms the foundation of herbal medicine, allowing practitioners to effectively tailor treatments to meet individual needs. Herbs can be used in various forms, such as teas, tinctures, poultices, and more, offering a versatile and natural approach to health and wellness. However, it's important to consult with a knowledgeable herbalist or healthcare provider before using herbs, especially for medicinal purposes, to ensure safety and efficacy.

It is worth noting that herbs can possess multiple actions, meaning they can have various effects on the body. For instance, chamomile is both a nervine, calming the nervous system, and an anti-inflammatory, reducing inflammation. This multifunctionality makes herbs versatile tools in herbal medicine.

The Concept of Energetics in Herbalism
Energetics in herbalism refer to the qualities of herbs that affect their interactions with the body beyond their chemical constituents. This concept includes the "temperature" of herbs (hot, cold, warm, cool) and their "moisture" level (drying, moistening). Energetics help in selecting herbs based on an individual's constitution and specific health needs.

For example, a person with a "cold" constitution might benefit from "warming" herbs like ginger or cinnamon, while someone with "hot" conditions might find relief with "cooling" herbs like peppermint or chamomile. Similarly, "dry" conditions can be balanced with "moistening" herbs like marshmallow root, and "wet" conditions might be addressed with "drying" herbs like sage.

Indigenous cultures have long understood these principles, often integrating them into their healing practices. They have traditionally recognized the importance of balancing the body's internal environment with the external conditions and the properties of herbs. This holistic approach acknowledges the interconnectedness of all aspects of health, including physical, emotional, and spiritual well-being.

Anti-Nausea Herbs
Benefit: Help alleviate nausea and morning sickness, particularly during early pregnancy.
Ginger (Zingiber officinale)
Peppermint (Mentha piperita)
Chamomile (Matricaria chamomilla)
Wild Yam (Dioscorea villosa)

Astringents
Benefit: Tone and tighten tissues, which can be beneficial in managing minor bleeding or postpartum recovery.
Witch Hazel (Hamamelis virginiana)
Yarrow (Achillea millefolium)
Red Raspberry Leaf (Rubus idaeus)
Katrafay Bark (Cedrelopsis grevei)

Calmatives
Benefit: Promote calmness and reduce anxiety, aiding in relaxation and emotional well-being.
Lavender (Lavandula angustifolia)
Valerian (Valeriana officinalis)
Skullcap (Scutellaria lateriflora)

Digestive Aids
Benefit: Relieve digestive issues such as nausea, bloating, and gas, and support healthy digestion.
Fennel (Foeniculum vulgare)
Peppermint (Mentha piperita)
Dandelion Root (Taraxacum officinale)
Ginger (Zingiber officinale)

Diuretics
Benefit: Manage water retention and support urinary tract health.
Dandelion Leaf (Taraxacum officinale)
Nettle (Urtica dioica)
Corn Silk (Zea mays)

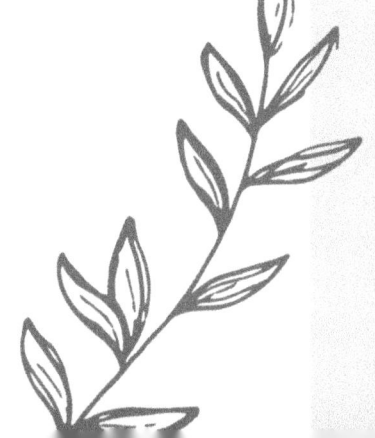

Galactagogues
Benefit: Support and increase milk production in breastfeeding mothers.
Fenugreek (Trigonella foenum-graecum)
Blessed Thistle (Cnicus benedictus)
Fennel (Foeniculum vulgare)
Goat's Rue (Galega officinalis)

Heart Openers
Benefit: Support emotional well-being and help manage postpartum emotions.
Hawthorn (Crataegus spp.)
Rose (Rosa spp.)
Motherwort (Leonurus cardiaca)

Immune Modulators
Benefit: Support and balance the immune system during pregnancy and postpartum.
Echinacea (Echinacea spp.)
Astragalus (Astragalus membranaceus)
Elderberry (Sambucus nigra)
Reishi Mushroom (Ganoderma lucidum)

Iron Builders
Benefit: Support healthy iron levels to prevent anemia, especially during pregnancy and postpartum.
Nettle (Urtica dioica)
Yellow Dock (Rumex crispus)
Dandelion Leaf (Taraxacum officinale)
Spirulina (Arthrospira platensis)

Nervines
Benefit: Support the nervous system, manage stress and anxiety, and promote relaxation.
Oat Straw (Avena sativa)
Chamomile (Matricaria chamomilla)
Skullcap (Scutellaria lateriflora)

Tonics
Benefit: Strengthen and support the body's systems, improving overall vitality and stamina.
Red Raspberry Leaf (Rubus idaeus)
Nettle (Urtica dioica)
Ashwagandha (Withania somnifera) postpartum only
Holy Basil (Ocimum sanctum)

Uterine Tonics for Labor
Benefit: Support uterine health and function, potentially aiding in labor and postpartum recovery.
Red Raspberry Leaf (Rubus idaeus)
Partridge Berry (Mitchella repens)

Vulnerary
Benefit: Aid in wound healing and tissue repair during postpartum recovery.
Calendula (Calendula officinalis)
Comfrey (Symphytum officinale)
Plantain (Plantago major)
Yarrow (Achillea millefolium)
Papaya (Carica papaya)

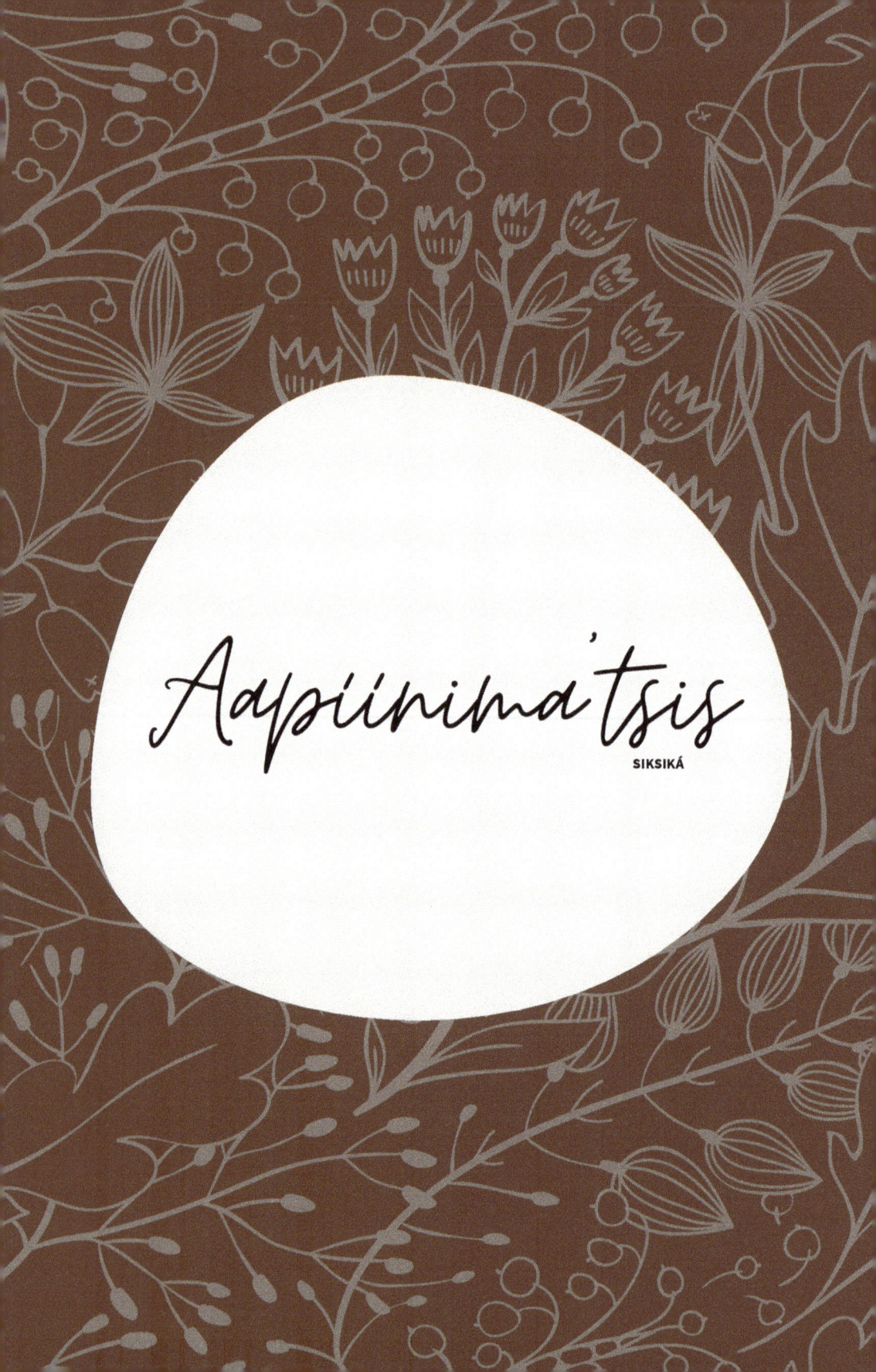

chapter 3

What to Avoid During Pregnancy

HERBS TO AVOID DURING PREGNANCY

Abortifacients

PENNYROYAL, RUE, TANSY, COTTON ROOT, WORMWOOD

Emmenagogues

ANGELICA, MUGWORT PENNYROYAL, RUE SAFFLOWER, SCOTCH BROOM, TANSY, THUJA WORMWOOD, YARROW

Teratogens

HEMLOCK
JIMSONWEED
GIANT FENNEL
TOBACCO
RAGWORT
NIGHTSHADE
CORN LILY

Stimulating Laxatives

ALOE
BUCKTHORN
CASCARA SAGRADA
CASTOR OIL
RHUBARB

Stimulants / Depressants

COFFEE
EPHEDRA
GUARANA

KAVA KAVA
PASSIONFLOWER

Alkaloids

BARBERRY
BORAGE
COLTSFOOT
COMFREY
GOLDENSEAL
OREGON GRAPE
KRATOM

Phytoestrogens

HOPS ISOFLAVONE
EXTRACTS RED CLOVER

Essential / Volatile Oils

OREGANO
PENNYROYAL
PEPPERMINT SAGE
TANSY
THUJA
THYME

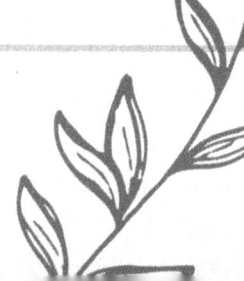

Emmenagogues

Emmenagogues are herbs that promote blood flow towards the pelvic area and uterus, and they can stimulate menstruation. These herbs are commonly used in cases of delayed or irregular menstrual cycles. Traditional and Indigenous cultures have long utilized emmenagogues for various health purposes, including managing menstrual health, addressing hormonal imbalances, and supporting the body's natural processes. Because emmenagogues stimulate the downward flow of blood and energy, they should be strictly avoided during pregnancy, as they may increase the risk of complications and loss.

Some well-known emmenagogues include:
1. Angelica (Angelica archangelica) - Often used to stimulate menstrual flow and relieve menstrual cramps.
2. Mugwort (Artemisia vulgaris) - Known for its ability to stimulate menstruation and regulate the menstrual cycle.
3. Pennyroyal Essential Oil (Mentha pulegium) - Used in very small quantities to encourage menstrual flow; caution advised due to potential toxicity.
4. Rue (Ruta graveolens) - Traditionally used to stimulate menstruation and relieve menstrual discomfort.
5. Safflower (Carthamus tinctorius) - Employed in some traditions to promote menstrual flow and support reproductive health.
6. Scotch Broom (Cytisus scoparius) - Used in certain herbal practices to promote menstruation and support uterine health.
7. Tansy (Tanacetum vulgare) - Known for its emmenagogue properties and traditionally used to stimulate menstrual flow.
8. Thuja (Thuja occidentalis) - Occasionally used to regulate menstrual cycles and support reproductive health.
9. Wormwood (Artemisia absinthium) - Utilized in herbal medicine to stimulate menstrual flow and address menstrual irregularities.
10. Yarrow (Achillea millefolium) - Employed to promote menstrual flow, ease menstrual cramps, and support overall menstrual health.
11. Blue Cohosh (Caulophyllum thalictroides): Used by Native American tribes, blue cohosh has been employed to stimulate labor and manage menstrual issues. However, its use requires caution due to potential toxicity.

In many Indigenous traditions, emmenagogues are not only used for their physical effects but also hold spiritual significance. They are sometimes part of rituals or ceremonies related to fertility, womanhood, and the cycles of nature. For example:

Mugwort (Artemisia vulgaris): In some Native American tribes, mugwort is burned as a smudge during ceremonies to honor the transition of girls into womanhood. It is believed to help in connecting with the spiritual realm and enhancing intuitive abilities. In Traditional Chinese Medicine, mugwort is used in moxibustion, where it is burned near the skin to stimulate energy flow, particularly during menstrual and reproductive health treatments.

Yarrow (Achillea millefolium): In Celtic traditions, yarrow was used in rituals to bless women entering puberty or motherhood. It was believed to protect against negative influences and promote healing. Yarrow was also used as a charm in love spells and fertility rites.

Motherwort (Leonurus cardiaca): In European folk traditions, motherwort was considered a protective herb for women, especially during childbirth. It was often included in amulets or burned in rituals to promote a safe delivery and postpartum recovery.

Red Clover (Trifolium pratense): Among Indigenous peoples in North America, red clover has been used in ceremonies to purify and bless women before marriage or childbirth. The herb's association with fertility and abundance made it a symbol of prosperity and good fortune.

Calendula (Calendula officinalis): In Mexican and other Latin American traditions, calendula is used in Day of the Dead (Día de los Muertos) ceremonies. While not strictly an emmenagogue, its flowers are believed to guide the spirits of the departed back to their families. In a broader sense, calendula's use in rituals symbolizes the cycles of life and death, akin to the menstrual and reproductive cycles.

These examples illustrate that emmenagogues are not merely medicinal but also hold deep cultural and spiritual meanings. They are often used to mark significant life transitions, connect with ancestors, and invoke blessings and protection. The rituals surrounding these herbs emphasize the interconnectedness of physical, emotional, and spiritual health.

Abortifacients

Abortifacients are herbs that may induce miscarriage or spontaneous abortion. Due to the high risk of toxicity and potential harm, including damage to the kidneys and liver, these herbs should be entirely avoided during pregnancy. Historically, abortifacients have been used in various cultures, often in situations where modern medical options were unavailable. They were used under the guidance of knowledgeable herbalists or traditional healers, who understood the risks and potential consequences. Some herbs traditionally known for their abortifacient properties include:
Pennyroyal (Mentha pulegium): Used in European and Native American traditions, pennyroyal has been known to induce menstruation and, in higher doses, abortion. However, it is highly toxic and can cause severe liver and kidney damage.

Tansy (Tanacetum vulgare): Employed in European folk medicine, tansy was used to induce abortion and expel retained tissues. It contains toxic compounds that can be dangerous.
Rue (Ruta graveolens): Used in Mediterranean cultures, rue has been used for its emmenagogue and abortifacient properties. It requires extreme caution due to its potential toxicity.
Cotton Root Bark (Gossypium herbaceum): Used by enslaved African women in the Americas, cotton root bark was a traditional abortifacient. It was sometimes used in desperate situations where access to other reproductive healthcare was denied.
In many Indigenous and traditional cultures, the use of abortifacients was often intertwined with spiritual practices and beliefs. The decision to use such herbs was not taken lightly, and the guidance of experienced healers was crucial. Today, it is important to approach the historical use of these herbs with respect for the cultural context and an understanding of the risks involved.

In contemporary herbalism, it is crucial to prioritize safety and consult with qualified professionals particularly when dealing with abortifacients. These herbs, while historically and culturally significant, carry potent effects that can pose serious health risks if misused. The use of these herbs should be approached with extreme caution due to the potential for toxicity and adverse health outcomes. One of the significant dangers associated with the improper use of abortifacient herbs is the risk of partial abortions. This condition occurs when the herbs fail to expel all the contents of the uterus, leading to retained tissue. Partial abortions can cause severe complications, such as infection, hemorrhaging, and the need for surgical intervention. The risk of incomplete abortion and subsequent complications underscores the necessity of having these procedures overseen by a trained and experienced practitioner who can manage any issues that may arise. Additionally, many of these herbs can be toxic, particularly at higher doses. For example, pennyroyal, rue, and tansy contain compounds that can cause liver and kidney damage, severe gastrointestinal distress, cardiovascular issues, and disruption of normal hormonal balance convulsions, and even death, if not used correctly. While the historical and cultural uses of abortifacients are rich and complex, modern application must be grounded in a thorough understanding of their potential risks. This careful and respectful approach helps to honor the traditional knowledge while prioritizing the safety and well-being of those seeking herbal remedies.

Teratogen

Teratogens are substances that can disturb the development of an embryo or fetus, potentially leading to birth defects or pregnancy loss. Always remember T = Toxic when it comes to teratogens. They encompass a wide range of agents, including radiation, certain medications, recreational drugs, tobacco products, chemicals, alcohol, specific infections, and even some health conditions like uncontrolled diabetes in pregnant people.

In various traditional and Indigenous cultures, awareness of teratogens has shaped pregnancy practices and guidelines, often woven into cultural beliefs and taboos.
Radiation and Environmental Exposures: Some Indigenous cultures have traditional practices to protect pregnant women from harmful environmental exposures. For example, certain Native American tribes advise avoiding specific areas or activities considered spiritually or physically dangerous during pregnancy.

Medications and Herbal Remedies: Traditional healers often recognize the potential dangers of certain substances during pregnancy. In Traditional Chinese Medicine, potent herbs are avoided due to their strong effects, which could harm the developing fetus.

Recreational Drugs and Tobacco: Many traditional medical practices discourage the use of substances like tobacco, particularly for pregnant women. Indigenous communities in North America have long understood the harmful effects of tobacco and traditionally use it in controlled, ritualistic ways.

Alcohol: Many cultures have specific rituals or taboos surrounding alcohol consumption, particularly for pregnant women. Expectant mothers are often advised to abstain from ingesting alcohol, and its use in ceremonies is generally controlled and regulated.

Infections and Disease: Certain infections are acknowledged as dangerous during pregnancy. In traditional African medicine, there are specific practices and herbal treatments to prevent infections like malaria, recognizing the risks they pose to both mother and fetus.

These cultural practices and beliefs highlight a community's efforts to protect the health of pregnant individuals and their unborn children, demonstrating a holistic understanding of health that encompasses both visible and invisible dangers. This traditional wisdom plays a crucial role in supporting healthy pregnancies and preventing harm to the developing fetus.

Phytoestrogens

Phytoestrogens are plant-based compounds that can mimic or modulate estrogen activity in the body. They can have both estrogenic (mimicking estrogen) and antiestrogenic (blocking estrogen) effects, depending on the context and the individual's hormonal balance. During pregnancy, excessive intake of phytoestrogens may lead to endocrine disruption, potentially causing developmental issues in the fetus. For example, they might contribute to early puberty, irregular menstrual cycles, and fertility problems in female babies, and an increased incidence of urological birth defects in male babies.

It is essential to approach phytoestrogens with caution during pregnancy. Eating naturally occurring phytoestrogens, such as those found in chickpeas, sunflower seeds, lentils, flaxseeds, soy products, and certain fruits and vegetables, in moderation as part of a balanced diet is generally considered safe. However, it is crucial to avoid consuming these compounds in medically impactful amounts, such as through concentrated supplements or high doses of specific phytoestrogen-rich herbs.

1. Red Clover (Trifolium pratense): Contains isoflavones, which are a type of phytoestrogen.
2. Black Cohosh (Cimicifuga racemosa): Contains phytoestrogenic compounds and is often used for menopausal symptoms.
3. Dong Quai (Angelica sinensis): Known as "female ginseng," it contains compounds that may mimic estrogen.
4. Licorice Root (Glycyrrhiza glabra): Contains isoflavonoids that have estrogenic effects.
5. Hops (Humulus lupulus): Contains 8-prenylnaringenin, a potent phytoestrogen.
6. Soy (Glycine max): Rich in isoflavones, especially genistein and daidzein.
7. Alfalfa (Medicago sativa): Contains coumestans, which are a type of phytoestrogen.

Stimulants

Stimulants increase risk of preeclampsia and preterm birth during pregnancy. Their use during the first trimester also increased the risk of placental abruption. One question often asked is the safety of caffeine. Consuming large amounts of caffeine during pregnancy may increase the risk of miscarriage or low birthweight, so it is best to limit the intake of caffeine.

If pregnant, limit caffeine to 200 milligrams each day. This is about the amount in one 12-ounce cup of coffee. If breastfeeding, limit caffeine to no more than two cups of coffee a day. For an energy boost during pregnancy, there are herbal alternatives to coffee that avoid the risks of caffeine. While generally considered safe, it is important to use them in moderation and consult your healthcare provider if you have any concerns.

1. Rooibos and Ginseng Tea: While rooibos itself is caffeine-free and calming, adding a small amount of ginseng (specifically Panax ginseng) can provide a gentle, energizing effect. However, ginseng should be used in moderation and with caution during pregnancy, so consult with a healthcare provider before consumption.
2. Guayusa Tea: This Amazonian leaf is rich in antioxidants . It has caffeine, but in lower amounts than coffee. it is known for providing sustained energy without the jitters often associated with coffee.
3. Maca Root Powder: Often added to smoothies, maca root is an adaptogen that can help boost energy levels and stamina. It is a phytoestrogen; however, in culinary amounts it is considered safe.
4. Schisandra Berries: Known for their adaptogenic properties, schisandra berries can help improve concentration and combat fatigue. They can be made into a tea or added to smoothies.
5. Yerba Maté (in moderation): Yerba maté contains natural caffeine and other compounds that can provide an energy boost. Consume it in moderation as the caffeine content may still be a concern during pregnancy.
6. Ginger and Turmeric Tea: While ginger is often associated with calming nausea, both ginger and turmeric can also provide an energizing effect.
7. Coconut Water with Spirulina: Coconut water is hydrating and contains natural electrolytes, and spirulina, a nutrient-dense algae, can provide a natural energy boost. This combination can be consumed as a refreshing drink that helps combat fatigue.
8. Beetroot Juice: Beetroot juice is rich in nitrates, which can improve blood flow and energy levels. it is a great natural pick-me-up that can be consumed on its own or added to smoothies.
9. Matcha (in moderation): Matcha green tea contains a moderate amount of caffeine and L-theanine, an amino acid that can promote calm alertness. Like yerba maté, it should be consumed in moderation and with professional guidance during pregnancy.

Lucuma Powder: A natural sweetener with a subtle caramel taste, it can be added to smoothies or hot drinks. It contains natural sugars and nutrients that can provide a gentle energy boost.

Depressants

The use of depressants during pregnancy can lead to miscarriage (especialy during the first trimester), birth defects, premature babies, underweight babies, and stillborn births. The more depressants ingested, the the higher the risks. Some depressants pass from the blood through the placenta and into the baby.

A baby's liver is one of the last organs to develop and does not mature until the later stages of pregnancy. It cannot process toxins well and too much exposure can significantly impact fetal development. Once born, the baby may have distinct facial features, demonstrate poor growth, and may exhibit learning and behavioural problems.

Some herbs have depressant effects and should be avoided during pregnancy due to their potential to harm the developing fetus. These include:

1. Kava (Piper methysticum) - Known for its calming effects, kava can act as a depressant and may affect fetal development.
2. Passionflower (Passiflora incarnata) - Though often used to relieve anxiety and insomnia, passionflower can have depressant effects.

Safe Herbal Alternatives to Depressants During Pregnancy
1. Chamomile (Matricaria chamomilla) - Calming and can help with relaxation and sleep.
2. Lavender (Lavandula angustifolia) - Soothing scent useful in aromatherapy for stress relief.
3. Lemon Balm (Melissa officinalis) - Mildly calming, helps alleviate anxiety and improves mood.
4. Holy Basil (Ocimum sanctum) - Adaptogenic herb that helps manage stress and balance mood.
5. Skullcap (Scutellaria lateriflora) - Calming herb that supports relaxation and reduces anxiety.

Laxatives

Constipation is a common pregnancy complaint but pregnant people must use caution when reaching for laxatives. They can remove nutrients from the mother's body before she has a chance to nourish the unborn baby or herself. A malnurished fetus may develop birth defects. Stimulating laxatives are especially concerning. They may induces contractions of the uterus and pelvic bleeding. This, in turn, may leads to a miscarriage. Safer alternatives include stool softeners, Safer alternatives include non-stimulating laxatives such as psyllium husk, yellow dock, marshmallow root, slippery elm, dandelion root, and flaxseed.

Alkaloids

An alkaloid is a large group of plant made chemicals that have nitrogen in them. Many alkaloids have a powerful pharmacologic impact. Certain alkaloids may be contraindicated during pregnancy because of their ability to disrupt fetal blood supply, which can lead to fetal damage, fetal dependency, or death. Kratom, berberine, sangunarine, mescaline, ephedrine, cocaine, nicotine, strychnine, methamphetamine are examples of alkaloids that have negative impacts during pregnancy.

Essential Oils & Volatile Oils

While some essential oils can be supportive of pregnancy there are certain oils that should be avoided. Use of essential oils in early pregnancy should be done with caution because they could potentially cause uterine contractions or adversely affect the baby in their early developmental stages. It is not recommended to ingest essential oils during pregnancy. Instead, use them on a cotton ball, in a diffuser, or to make a hydrosol. Some essentials that are supportive of pregnancy are cardamom and ginger which are useful during bouts of morning sickness. While chamomile, lavender, and frankincense can help with relaxation.

Essential Oils to Avoid During Pregnancy:
1. Clary Sage (except for during labor)
2. Rosemary
3. Peppermint (in high amounts)
4. Oregano
5. Thyme
6. Cinnamon
7. Basil
8. Wintergreen
9. Tansy
10. Pennyroyal

Certain chemical components found in plants can pose risks during pregnancy due to their potential effects on the mother and fetus. Here's a list of some of these components, along with examples of plants that contain them:

Thujone
Effects: Neurotoxic, can stimulate uterine contractions.
Found in: Wormwood (Artemisia absinthium), Sage (Salvia officinalis), Hyssop (Hyssopus officinalis).

Berberine
Effects: Can stimulate the uterus and affect fetal development.
Found in: Goldenseal (Hydrastis canadensis), Barberry (Berberis vulgaris), Oregon grape (Mahonia aquifolium).

Pyrrolizidine Alkaloids
Effects: Hepatotoxic, can cause liver damage and be harmful to the fetus.
Found in: Comfrey (Symphytum officinale), Coltsfoot (Tussilago farfara), Borage (Borago officinalis).

Anthraquinones
Effects: Strong laxatives, can cause uterine contractions.
Found in: Aloe (Aloe vera), Senna (Senna alexandrina), Rhubarb (Rheum rhabarbarum).

Safrole
Effects: Carcinogenic, hepatotoxic.
Found in: Sassafras (Sassafras albidum), Nutmeg (Myristica fragrans), Camphor (Cinnamomum camphora).

Essential Oils with Emmenagogue or Abortifacient Properties
Effects: Can stimulate menstruation or induce contractions.
Found in: Pennyroyal (Mentha pulegium), Mugwort (Artemisia vulgaris), Tansy (Tanacetum vulgare).

Isoquinoline Alkaloids
Effects: Potentially teratogenic, can affect fetal development.
Found in: Bloodroot (Sanguinaria canadensis), Poppy (Papaver somniferum).

Methyl Salicylate
Effects: Similar to aspirin, can cause bleeding issues.
Found in: Wintergreen (Gaultheria procumbens), Sweet Birch (Betula lenta).

Coumarins
Effects: Anticoagulant, can increase bleeding risk.
Found in: Tonka bean (Dipteryx odorata), Sweet clover (Melilotus officinalis).

Ergot Alkaloids
Effects: Can cause strong uterine contractions and potentially lead to miscarriage.
Found in: Ergot fungus (Claviceps purpurea).

This list includes some of the more well-known components and associated herbs that should be avoided during pregnancy. However, it is not exhaustive, and there are other herbs and components that may also be contraindicated.

"The land has wisdom; the land has teachings. And the herbs that grow upon it are not just commodities, but teachers, healers, and members of our community."

Leah Penniman
Co-Director of Soul Fire Farm

chapter 4

Tradition in Pregnancy Care
Botanical support for Pregnancy
Pregnancy Wellness Recipes
Pregnancy Cold & Flu Support
Botanical Support For Complex Pregnancy

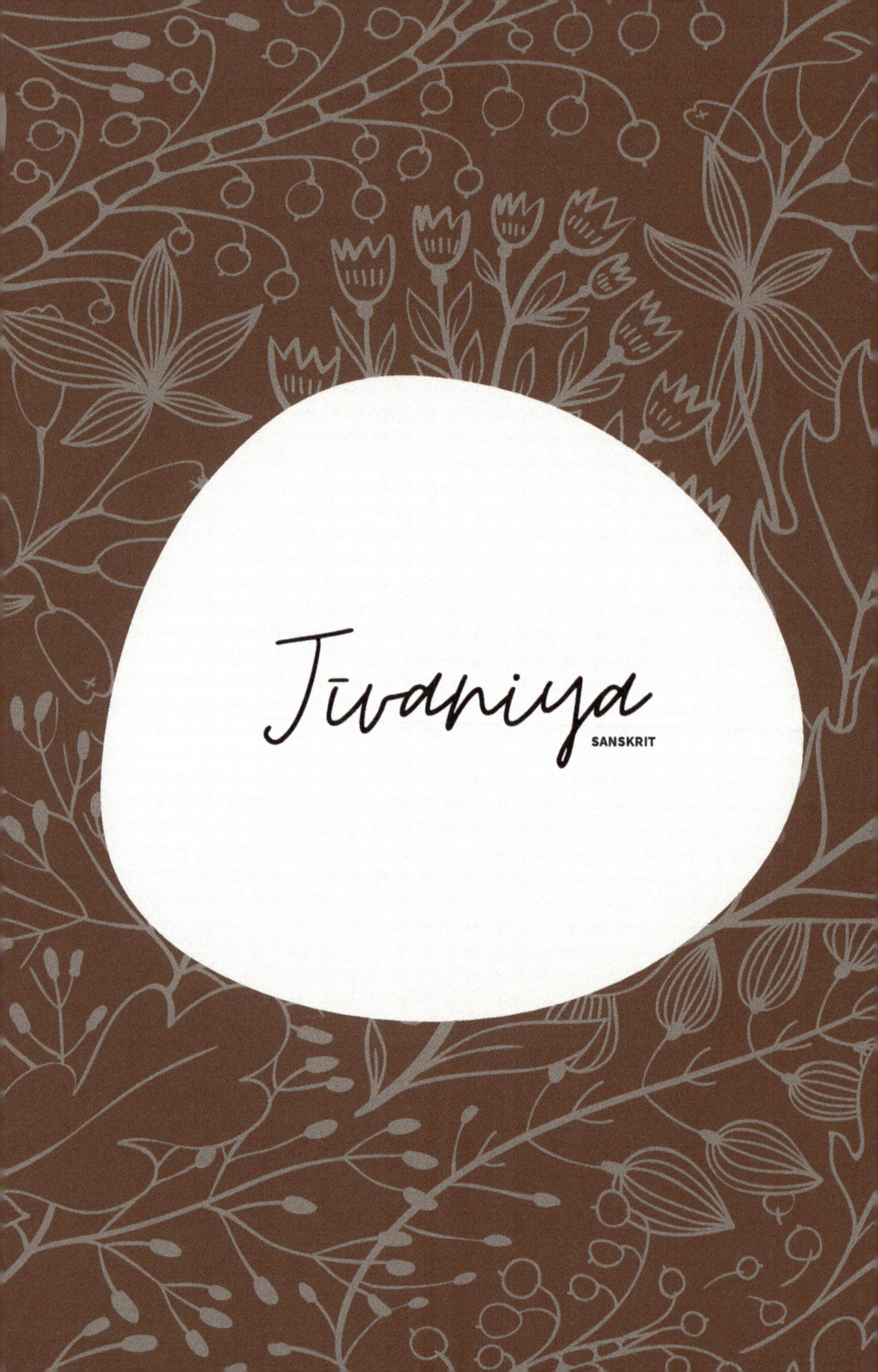

The Role of Tradition in Pregnancy Care

In many cultures, pregnancy is seen through a deeply holistic lens, integrating the physical, spiritual, and communal aspects of life. This perspective honors the profound connection between the expectant mother, the unborn child, and the natural world. Here, pregnancy is not just a personal journey but a communal event. The support network extends far beyond immediate family, embracing the entire community, which includes ancestors, elders, future children, and even plant relatives. This collective involvement is often expressed through rituals, ceremonies, and shared care practices designed to ensure the health and well-being of both mother and baby. These practices may involve offerings, prayers, and ceremonies to honor new life and seek blessings for a healthy pregnancy.

Herbs and plants play a crucial role in traditional pregnancy care. Various traditional medicine systems use plant-based remedies to support the health of the mother and child. Herbs are used to alleviate common pregnancy discomforts, support a healthy labor, and aid in postpartum recovery.

Balancing physical health with emotional and spiritual well-being is central to holistic care. Traditional practices may involve dietary adjustments, ample rest, and herbal remedies to nurture and support the mother's body. Emotional and mental health is also prioritized, with practices aimed at creating a supportive and peaceful environment for the mother.

Respecting the natural cycles and rhythms of the earth and body is essential. This respect extends to the cycle of pregnancy, viewed as a natural part of life's continuum. There's a strong emphasis on living in harmony with nature and aligning practices with the natural world, considering seasonal changes, lunar cycles, and other natural rhythms that influence health and well-being.

Indigenous perspectives on pregnancy are deeply rooted in tradition and knowledge passed down through elders and healers. This knowledge includes not only the use of medicinal plants but also cultural practices, stories, and rituals that support the journey of pregnancy and childbirth. The wisdom of these traditions is cherished and preserved as a vital part of cultural heritage.

In our globally connected time, we have the unique opportunity to learn from and support each other in ways never before possible. It is our duty to support the birthing community, as they are the portals to the next generation. A healthy birth that nurtures the mind, body, spirit, and baby lays the foundation for a successful and fulfilling journey into motherhood, ensuring a strong start for the future.

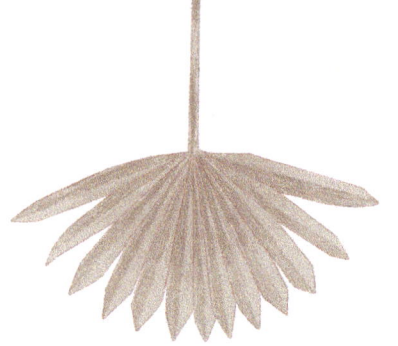

I have experienced three pregnancies and given birth to two beautiful children, with herbs playing a crucial role throughout each journey. These herbs were instrumental in helping me heal from loss, strengthening me for subsequent pregnancies, and providing comfort through common pregnancy discomforts rarely discussed, like constipation and severe digestive issues.

For my first birth, I was intensely focused on labor. I had imagined it as the grand finale of a marathon I'd been running for over nine months. I meticulously prepared with books, oils, a carefully curated soundtrack, and even a birthing gown. My planning might be described as a bit type A, but I quickly learned that babies don't adhere to plans or care about outfits. My labor lasted nearly 30 hours, and while the experience was challenging, I am profoundly grateful for the support system that surrounded me. This included the ancestors who guided me in dreams, my doula who supported me through each stage, my husband who helped me through contractions, my mother and mother-in-law who provided hands-on support, and my father who stood watchful guard. I am also deeply thankful for Dr. Viega, who assisted me through both births, and Dr. Angel, who provided vigilant care during my pregnancies, shielding me from unnecessary procedures and helping me trust in my body's abilities.

In my second pregnancy, I shifted my focus to postpartum support. I dedicated my research to creating a "golden month" of recovery, integrating herbs into my diet, steaming with them for 40 days post-birth, and using them to support my breast milk and overall healing. This approach allowed me to regain my vitality more quickly and provided valuable support during breastfeeding. Seeing the benefits of this method inspired me to help others curate their own golden month, guiding them in creating a supportive system through herbs, food, community, and ritual. I am committed to ensuring that every birthing person has the opportunity to support and heal themselves in a nurturing, personalized way.

With this experience and understanding in mind, I invite you to embrace a set of pregnancy affirmations that can guide and support you through this transformative time. These affirmations are crafted to help you connect with your inner strength, trust your body, and honor the sacred journey of pregnancy.

Pregnancy Affirmations

Find a comfortable position and close your eyes. Take a deep breath in, and as you exhale, let go of any tension.

Repeat these affirmations silently or aloud, letting their truth resonate within you:

"I trust in the wisdom of my body."
"I am connected to the strength of my ancestors."

I embrace the natural rhythm of my body and trust in its wisdom."
"My body knows how to nourish and bring forth new life."
"I am surrounded by love, guidance, and the energy of my ancestors."

"My baby has chosen me with love and purpose."
"I am capable, strong, and ready for this journey."
"I am resilient and capable of handling whatever comes my way."
"I am grounded, centered, and in tune with the sacred process of birth."
Feel the power of these words as they echo through your being. Know that you are supported, cherished, and prepared for the beautiful experience of bringing new life into the world.

When you are ready, gently bring your awareness back to the present moment. Take a few deep breaths and slowly open your eyes, carrying with you the strength, trust, and wisdom of this meditation.

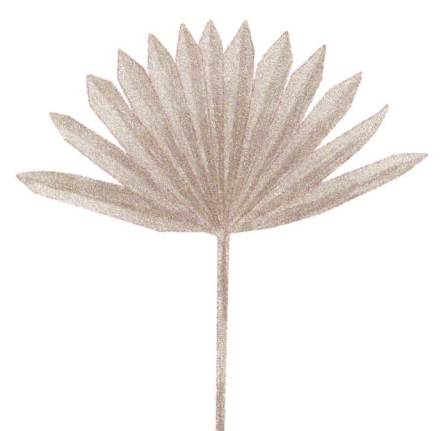

Botanical Support FOR PREGNANCY

ALFALFA
Medicago sativa
A NUTRITIOUS HERB THAT PROVIDES ESSENTIAL VITAMINS AND MINERALS, MAKING IT BENEFICIAL DURING PREGNANCY. IT IS RICH IN CALCIUM, IRON, AND VITAMIN K, WHICH SUPPORTS BONE HEALTH AND BLOOD CLOTTING. ALFALFA ALSO AIDS IN DIGESTION AND HELPS PREVENT ANEMIA BY IMPROVING IRON LEVELS. ITS GENTLE NATURE MAKES IT A SAFE AND SUPPORTIVE CHOICE FOR NOURISHING BOTH MOTHER AND BABY.

ALOE
Aloe vera
EXTERNAL USE ONLY; SOOTHES SKIN IRRITATIONS AND BURNS.

ASTRAGALUS
Astragalus membranaceus
KNOWN FOR ITS IMMUNE-MODULATING PROPERTIES, MAKING IT ESPECIALLY BENEFICIAL DURING PREGNANCY. IT HELPS SUPPORT THE BODY'S IMMUNE SYSTEM, PROMOTING OVERALL HEALTH AND RESILIENCE. DURING PREGNANCY, ASTRAGALUS CAN ASSIST IN ENHANCING VITALITY AND ENERGY LEVELS, IT ALSO HELPS IN STRENGTHENING THE BODY'S DEFENSES, PROVIDING ADDED SUPPORT DURING THE STRESSFUL PERIOD OF PREGNANCY AND RECOVERY.

BLACK HAW
Viburnum prunifolium
VALUED FOR ITS SUPPORTIVE ROLE DURING PREGNANCY. IT IS OFTEN USED TO HELP RELAX THE UTERUS AND EASE CRAMPS DURING LABOR. BLACK HAW MAY ALSO BE BENEFICIAL IN REDUCING IMPLANTATION PAIN AND MANAGING BLOOD PRESSURE, PROVIDING COMFORT AND SUPPORT THROUGHOUT PREGNANCY.

BURDOCK
Arctium lappa
BURDOCK IS KNOWN FOR ITS DETOXIFYING PROPERTIES AND SUPPORTIVE ROLE DURING PREGNANCY. IT PROMOTES HEALTHY SKIN, AIDS IN THE BODY'S CLEANSING PROCESSES, AND SUPPORTS LIVER FUNCTION, MAKING IT A VALUABLE HERB FOR OVERALL WELL-BEING.

CALENDULA
Calendula officinalis
CALENDULA IS A CALMING HERB THAT SUPPORTS SKIN HEALTH AND HEALING DURING PREGNANCY. IT IS OFTEN USED TOPICALLY TO SOOTHE INFLAMMATION

CHAMOMILE
Matricaria chamomilla
CHAMOMILE IS A SOOTHING HERB THAT SUPPORTS RELAXATION AND DIGESTIVE COMFORT DURING PREGNANCY. IT CAN BE USED INTERNALLY TO CALM NERVES AND EASE DIGESTIVE ISSUES, AS WELL AS TOPICALLY TO SOOTHE SKIN IRRITATIONS AND INFLAMMATION.

CHICKWEED
Stellaria media
KNOWN FOR ITS SOOTHING AND COOLING PROPERTIES, CHICKWEED CAN HELP ALLEVIATE ITCHING AND SKIN IRRITATIONS DURING PREGNANCY, PROMOTING COMFORT AND RELIEF. IT IS ALSO USED TO SUPPORT THE BODY'S NATURAL DETOXIFICATION PROCESSES AND CAN BE BENEFICIAL FOR SOOTHING DIGESTIVE DISCOMFORT.

CHAYA
Cnidoscolus aconitifolius
A LEAFY GREEN THAT IS RICH IN NUTRIENTS LIKE CALCIUM AND IRON, BENEFICIAL DURING PREGNANCY.

CINNAMON
Cinnamomum verum
IN MODERATION, CINNAMON CAN SUPPORT BLOOD FLOW, DIGESTION, INFLAMMATION RELIEF, IMMUNITY, AND HEALTHY BLOOD SUGAR DURING PREGNANCY, BUT EXCESSIVE AMOUNTS SHOULD BE AVOIDED DUE TO POTENTIAL RISKS OF UTERINE CONTRACTIONS.

COCONUT
Cocos nucifera

A HYDRATING AND NUTRITIOUS CHOICE FOR PREGNANT WOMEN. COCONUT WATER PROVIDES ELECTROLYTES FOR HYDRATION, WHILE COCONUT MEAT AND OIL OFFER HEALTHY FATS FOR FETAL DEVELOPMENT. IT IS GENTLE ON THE DIGESTIVE SYSTEM AND CAN SOOTHE PREGNANCY-RELATED NAUSEA.

DAMIANA
Turnera diffusa

USED IN PREGNANCY TO SUPPORT EMOTIONAL WELL-BEING AND RELIEVE STRESS. IT MAY ALSO ENHANCE MOOD AND PROMOTE A CALM, POSITIVE STATE OF MIND DURING PREGNANCY.

DANDELION RT
Taraxacum officinale

SUPPORTS PREGNANCY BY AIDING IN DIGESTION, RELIEVING WATER RETENTION, AND PROVIDING NUTRIENTS LIKE VITAMINS AND MINERALS. IT ALSO HELPS SUPPORT THE BODY'S DETOXIFICATION PROCESSES AND PROMOTES OVERALL WELL-BEING.

ECHINACEA
Echinacea angustifolia (or purpurea)

SUPPORTS PREGNANCY BY HELPING TO STRENGTHEN THE IMMUNE SYSTEM AND PROMOTE OVERALL HEALTH. IT IS USED TO SUPPORT GENERAL WELL-BEING AND HELP PREVENT ILLNESSES, MAKING IT A VALUABLE HERB FOR MAINTAINING VITALITY DURING PREGNANCY.

ELDER
Sambucus nigra

HELPS SUPPORT PREGNANCY BY PROVIDING GENTLE DIURETIC AND ANTI-INFLAMMATORY EFFECTS. IT MAY ALSO HELP RELIEVE MILD CONGESTION AND SUPPORT OVERALL COMFORT. ELDERBERRY ENHANCES IMMUNE FUNCTION AND OFFERS ANTIOXIDANT PROTECTION, SUPPORTING GENERAL HEALTH DURING PREGNANCY. IT CAN HELP STRENGTHEN THE BODY'S DEFENSES.

ELECAMPANE
Inula helenium

SUPPORTS RESPIRATORY HEALTH DURING PREGNANCY. KNOWN FOR ITS EXPECTORANT PROPERTIES, ELECAMPANE CAN HELP EASE COUGHS AND CLEAR MUCUS.

ELEUTHERO
Eleutherococcus senticosus

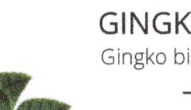

SUPPORTS OVERALL ENERGY AND STAMINA DURING PREGNANCY. KNOWN AS AN ADAPTOGEN, ELEUTHERO CAN HELP THE BODY ADAPT TO STRESS AND IMPROVE RESILIENCE.

GINGKO
Gingko biloba

ENHANCES CIRCULATION AND MAY SUPPORT MEMORY AND FOCUS DURING PREGNANCY. GENERALLY SAFE IN MODERATION

GINSENG
Panax ginseng

GINSENG IS KNOWN FOR ITS ADAPTOLITIC PROPERTIES, WHICH CAN HELP IMPROVE ENERGY AND RESILIENCE TO STRESS. USE IN MODERATION

GINGER
Zingiber offcinale

HELPS ALLEVIATE NAUSEA AND MORNING SICKNESS DURING PREGNANCY. IT ALSO OFFERS GENTLE DIGESTIVE SUPPORT AND CAN HELP REDUCE INFLAMMATION, PROMOTING OVERALL COMFORT

GOLDENROD Solidago spp	VALUED FOR ITS SUPPORTIVE ROLE IN URINARY HEALTH AND REDUCING INFLAMMATION. IT CAN HELP EASE DISCOMFORT AND PROMOTE HEALTHY KIDNEY FUNCTION DURING PREGNANCY.
HAWTHORNE Crataegus spp	KNOWN FOR SUPPORTING CIRCULATORY HEALTH AND STRENGTHENING THE HEART. DURING PREGNANCY, IT CAN HELP IMPROVE CIRCULATION AND SUPPORT OVERALL CARDIOVASCULAR WELL-BEING.
HOLY BASIL Ocimum sanctum	SUPPORTS STRESS RELIEF AND EMOTIONAL WELL-BEING DURING PREGNANCY. KNOWN FOR ITS ADAPTOGENIC PROPERTIES
HOPS Humulus lupulus	HOPS ARE KNOWN FOR THEIR CALMING PROPERTIES AND CAN HELP PROMOTE RELAXATION AND IMPROVE SLEEP QUALITY.
LEMON Citrus limon	PROVIDES VITAMIN C AND ANTIOXIDANTS, SUPPORTING IMMUNE FUNCTION AND OVERALL HEALTH DURING PREGNANCY. IT CAN HELP WITH DIGESTIVE COMFORT AND HYDRATION, AND ITS REFRESHING FLAVOR MAKES IT A POPULAR ADDITION TO FLUID INTAKE.
MACA Lepidium meyenii	MACA IS VALUED FOR ITS ENERGY-BOOSTING AND ADAPTOGENIC PROPERTIES. IT MAY HELP SUPPORT ENERGY LEVELS AND STAMINA DURING PREGNANCY.
MARSHMALLOW Althaea officinalis	MARSHMALLOW ROOT IS KNOWN FOR ITS SOOTHING AND MOISTURIZING PROPERTIES. IT MAY HELP RELIEVE DIGESTIVE DISCOMFORTS AND SUPPORT HYDRATION IN THE BODY.
MORINGA Moringa oleifera	MORINGA LEAVES ARE NUTRIENT-DENSE AND PROVIDE ESSENTIAL VITAMINS AND MINERALS. THEY MAY SUPPORT OVERALL HEALTH AND WELL-BEING DURING PREGNANCY.
MULLIEN Verbascum thapsus	KNOWN FOR ITS SOOTHING PROPERTIES AND MAY HELP SUPPORT RESPIRATORY HEALTH.
NETTLE Urtica dioica	VALUED FOR ITS NUTRIENT-DENSE PROFILE AND MAY HELP SUPPORT OVERALL PREGNANCY HEALTH. IT IS RICH IN VITAMINS AND MINERALS, INCLUDING IRON AND CALCIUM, WHICH ARE BENEFICIAL FOR BOTH MOTHER AND BABY.

PEACH
Prunus persica

TRADITIONALLY USED FOR SOOTHING DIGESTIVE ISSUES, PROVIDING ANTIOXIDANT PROTECTION, REDUCING INFLAMMATION, AND SUPPORTING RESPIRATORY HEALTH. IT ALSO HELPS WITH RELAXATION AND STRESS RELIEF, AND MAY BENEFIT SKIN HEALTH.

PLANTAIN
Musa spp.

PLANTAIN IS VALUED FOR ITS NUTRIENT DENSITY AND CAN SUPPORT PREGNANCY BY PROVIDING VITAMINS A, C, AND K, AS WELL AS MINERALS LIKE POTASSIUM AND CALCIUM. IT MAY HELP PROMOTE DIGESTIVE HEALTH AND RELIEVE CONSTIPATION. PLANTAIN ALSO HAS ANTI-INFLAMMATORY PROPERTIES THAT CAN SUPPORT GENERAL WELL-BEING DURING PREGNANCY.

RED RASPBERRY
Rubus idaeus

RED RASPBERRY LEAF IS COMMONLY USED DURING PREGNANCY TO SUPPORT UTERINE TONE AND STRENGTHEN THE UTERUS. IT MAY HELP EASE LABOR BY PROMOTING EFFICIENT CONTRACTIONS AND SUPPORT POSTPARTUM RECOVERY. THIS HERB IS RICH IN VITAMINS AND MINERALS, INCLUDING VITAMINS C AND E, CALCIUM, AND MAGNESIUM, WHICH CAN CONTRIBUTE TO OVERALL MATERNAL HEALTH.

ROSE
Rosa spp.

ROSE IS VALUED FOR ITS CALMING AND MOISTURIZING PROPERTIES DURING PREGNANCY. IT CAN HELP ALLEVIATE ANXIETY, SUPPORT EMOTIONAL WELL-BEING, AND PROMOTE RELAXATION. ROSE PETALS ARE OFTEN USED IN TEAS OR TOPICALLY TO SOOTHE SKIN AND PROVIDE HYDRATION, WHICH CAN BE BENEFICIAL FOR STRETCH MARKS AND DRYNESS DURING PREGNANCY.

SKULLCAP
Scutellaria lateriflora

KNOWN FOR ITS CALMING AND RELAXING PROPERTIES. IT CAN HELP EASE NERVOUS TENSION AND PROMOTE BETTER SLEEP, WHICH CAN BE PARTICULARLY USEFUL DURING PREGNANCY. IT SUPPORTS OVERALL RELAXATION WITHOUT CAUSING DROWSINESS, MAKING IT A VALUABLE HERB FOR MANAGING STRESS AND ANXIETY.

SPIRULINA
Arthrospira platensis (or maxima)

SPIRULINA IS A NUTRIENT-DENSE ALGA THAT PROVIDES A RICH SOURCE OF PROTEIN, VITAMINS, AND MINERALS. IT SUPPORTS OVERALL NUTRITIONAL HEALTH DURING PREGNANCY, HELPING TO FILL NUTRIENT GAPS AND PROMOTE ENERGY LEVELS. ITS HIGH IRON CONTENT CAN ALSO BE BENEFICIAL FOR MAINTAINING HEALTHY BLOOD LEVELS.

TURMERIC
Curcuma longa

KNOWN FOR ITS ANTI-INFLAMMATORY AND ANTIOXIDANT PROPERTIES, WHICH CAN BE BENEFICIAL DURING PREGNANCY. IT SUPPORTS OVERALL HEALTH AND MAY HELP REDUCE INFLAMMATION IN THE BODY. TURMERIC CAN ALSO PROMOTE DIGESTIVE HEALTH AND SUPPORT IMMUNE FUNCTION.

WILD YAM
Dioscorea villosa

WILD YAM IS KNOWN FOR ITS POTENTIAL TO SUPPORT HORMONAL BALANCE DURING PREGNANCY. IT IS THOUGHT TO HELP EASE DISCOMFORTS ASSOCIATED WITH HORMONAL CHANGES

YELLOWDOCK
Rumex crispus

YELLOW DOCK IS KNOWN FOR ITS POTENTIAL TO SUPPORT DIGESTIVE HEALTH AND NUTRIENT ABSORPTION. DURING PREGNANCY, IT MAY BE USED TO HELP WITH CONSTIPATION AND TO SUPPORT OVERALL NUTRIENT INTAKE.

PREGNANCY WELLNESS RECIPES

ANEMIA

MAINTAINING ADEQUATE IRON LEVELS DURING PREGNANCY IS CRUCIAL FOR SUPPORTING THE INCREASED BLOOD VOLUME AND ENSURING SUFFICIENT OXYGEN SUPPLY TO BOTH THE MOTHER AND THE DEVELOPING BABY.

HERBS/REMEDIES: IRON RICH FOODS: BEETS AND LEAFY GREENS, NETTLE LEAF, DANDELION LEAF, ALFALAFA, AND SPIRULINA

CLEO'S GREEN COCO JUICE:
ADD 1 TBL OF SPIRULINA TO 8 OZ OF CHILLED COCONUT WATER. SHAKE AND ENJOY.

HEAVY NETTLE TINCTURE:
1 CUP DRIED NETTLE LEAVES
APPLE CIDER VINEGAR (ENOUGH TO COVER THE NETTLE LEAVES)
HONEY (OPTIONAL, TO TASTE)
JUICE OF 1 LEMON
*SEE TINCTURE INSTRUCTIONS IN HERBAL PREPERATIONS

CONSTIPATION TEA

CONSTIPATION DURING PREGNANCY OFTEN OCCURS DUE TO HORMONAL CHANGES THAT RELAX THE INTESTINAL MUSCLES, COMBINED WITH THE PRESSURE OF THE GROWING UTERUS ON THE INTESTINES, SLOWING DOWN DIGESTION. STIMULATING LAXATIVES ARE CONTRAINDICATED DURING PREGNANCY. THIS BLEND IS FORMULATED TO BE A GENTLE AND NUTRITIVE APPROACH TO ENCOURAGING BOWEL MOVEMENTS. USE IN MODERATION.

HERBS/REMEDIES: HYDRATION, HIGH FIBER FOODS, PSYLLIUM HUSK, YELLOWDOCK, GINGER

BIG BELLY TEA:
2 PARTS DANDELION ROOT
1 PART YELLOW DOCK
1 PART BURDOCK ROOT
1 PART SLIPPERY ELM
¼ PART GINGER

USE 1 TBL OF MIXTURE TO 1 CUP OF COLD WATER AND BRING TO SIMMER OVER LOW HEAT FOR 15 MINUTES. REMOVE FROM HEAT AND LET IT STEEP FOR 20 MINUTES TO OVERNIGHT. DRINK A CUP IN THE EVENING BEFORE BED..

EDEMA

EDEMA DURING PREGNANCY IS COMMON AND OCCURS DUE TO INCREASED BLOOD VOLUME AND PRESSURE FROM THE GROWING UTERUS, WHICH CAN CAUSE FLUID RETENTION IN THE BODY'S TISSUES.

HERBS/REMEDIES: ELECTROLYTES THAT ARE SALT NOT SUGAR BASED, GINGER FOR CIRCULATION, NETTLE, DANDELION LEAF

FLUID AND FLOW TEA:
1 PART NETTLE
½ PART CORNSILK
¼ PART DANDELION LEAF
¼ PART SPEARMINT

POUR BOILING WATER OVER DRIED OR FRESH HERBS, COVER, AND LET STEEP FOR 15-20 MINUTES. STRAIN AND ENJOY..

FATIGUE

FATIGUE DURING PREGNANCY IS OFTEN CAUSED BY HORMONAL CHANGES, INCREASED ENERGY DEMANDS OF THE BODY, AND THE PHYSICAL AND EMOTIONAL ADJUSTMENTS TO PREGNANCY.
HERBS AND REMEDIES: ADAPTOGENIC HERBS LIKE GINSENG, MACA, ELEUTHERO, RHODIOLA. SUPPORTIVE TONICS LIKE NETTLE AND ALFALFA, AND STIMULATING HERBS LIKE ROOIBOS AND PEPPERMINT

VITALI-TEA *(WORKS AS A SYRUP OR TINCTURE AS WELL).*
  1 PART ELEUTHERO
  ½ PART GINSENG
  ½ PART MACA
  ¼ PART CAROB

USE 1 TBL OF MIXTURE TO 1 CUP OF COLD WATER AND BRING TO SIMMER OVER LOW HEAT FOR 15 MINUTES.
REMOVE FROM HEAT AND LET IT STEEP FOR 20 MINUTES TO OVERNIGHT

HEART BURN

HEARTBURN DURING PREGNANCY IS COMMONLY CAUSED BY HORMONAL CHANGES THAT RELAX THE VALVE BETWEEN THE STOMACH AND ESOPHAGUS, ALONG WITH THE GROWING UTERUS PRESSING ON THE STOMACH, LEADING TO ACID REFLUX.

HERBS AND REMEDIES: SLIPPERY ELM AND MARSHMALLOW ROOT. ALSO SLEEP ELEVATED AND AVOID TRIGGERING FOODS LIKE SPICY FOODS.

CALM & SOOTHE BREW:
  1 PART SLIPPERY ELM
  1 PART MARSHMALLOW ROOT
  ½ PART CHAMOMILE

USE 1 TBL OF MIXTURE TO 1 CUP BOILED HOT WATER AND LET INFUSE FOR 10 MINUTES TO OVERNIGHT.
THE RESULTING TEA WILL BE VISCOUS LIKE A SYRUP

HEMMORHOID

HEMORRHOIDS DURING PREGNANCY ARE CAUSED BY INCREASED PRESSURE ON THE VEINS IN THE PELVIC AREA, OFTEN DUE TO THE GROWING UTERUS AND CHANGES IN BLOOD FLOW, LEADING TO SWELLING AND DISCOMFORT IN THE RECTAL AREA.

HERBS AND REMEDIES: STAY HYDRATED, ANTI-INFLAMMATORY FOODS AND HERBS, HEALTHY FATS, SEA MOSS,

ALOE SOOTHING GEL
  2 TBL ALOE VERA GEL (FRESH OR PURE, FROM THE PLANT OR STORE-BOUGHT)
  1 TBL WITCH HAZEL EXTRACT
  1 TBL CALENDULA OIL OR INFUSED CALENDULA OIL
  1 TSP VITAMIN E OIL (OPTIONAL FOR EXTRA SOOTHING)

IN A CLEAN BOWL, COMBINE THE ALOE VERA GEL, WITCH HAZEL EXTRACT, CALENDULA OIL, AND VITAMIN E OIL MIX WELL UNTIL FULLY COMBINED.
GENTLY APPLY A THIN LAYER OF THE MIXTURE TO THE AFFECTED AREA. USE CLEAN HANDS OR A COTTON PAD TO AVOID ANY IRRITATION.
FREQUENCY: APPLY 2-3 TIMES DAILY, ESPECIALLY AFTER BOWEL MOVEMENTS, OR AS NEEDED FOR RELIEF.
STORE: KEEP ANY LEFTOVER OINTMENT IN A SMALL, AIRTIGHT CONTAINER. STORE IN A COOL, DRY PLACE.

PREGNANCY WELLNESS RECIPES

PREGNANCY WELLNESS RECIPES

INSOMNIA

INSOMNIA DURING PREGNANCY CAN OCCUR DUE TO PHYSICAL DISCOMFORT, HORMONAL CHANGES, AND THE ANTICIPATION OF CHILDBIRTH, MAKING IT DIFFICULT FOR EXPECTANT MOTHERS TO GET RESTFUL SLEEP.

REST WELL TEA
- ½ PART HOLY BASIL
- ½ PART SKULLCAP
- ¼ PART NETTLE LEAF
- ¼ PART VALERIAN
- ¼ PART OAT TOPS
- ¼ PART CHAMOMILE

USE 1 TBL OF MIXTURE TO 1 CUP BOILED HOT WATER AND LET INFUSE FOR 10 MINUTES TO OVERNIGHT.

MORNING SICKNESS

THIS RECIPE WAS INSPIRED BY ROSEMARY GLADSTAR'S BOOK, "HEALING FOR WOMEN"

WILD YAM TINCTURE
- 1 PART WILD YAM ROOT
- 1 PARTDANDELION ROOT
- ½ PART GINGER ROOT

TAKE ¼ TSP THREE TIMES A DAY.
MAY BE TAKEN FREQUENTLY THROUGHOUT THE DAY DURING ACUTE BOUTS OF MORING SICKNESS.
*SEE TINCTURE INSTRUCTIONS IN HERBAL PREPERATIONS

LIMON Y SAL
THIS RECIPE COMES FROM MY MOTHER AND IS COMMON REMEDY FOR NAUSEA IN PUERTO RICO.

WASH THE OUTSIDE OF A LEMON, SLICE IT, AND SPRINKLE IT WITH SALT. WHENEVER YOU BEGING TO FILL NAUSEATED , SUCK THE SALTY CITRUS JUICE AND CHEW ON THE BITTER RIND.

PEACH LEAF TEA
THIS REMEDY CAME FROM THE TRADITONS OF SOUTHERN BLACK MIDWIVES.

- 1 PART PEACH LEAVES
- 2 PARTS SPEARMINT LEAF
- ½ PART FRESH GRATED GINGER ROOT

USE 1 TO 2 TBL OF LEAVES PER CUP OF WATER.
ADD TO COLD WATER AND BRING TO A SIMMER OVER LOW HEAT.
REMOVE FROM HEAT AND LET STEEP FOR 20 MINUTES TO OVERNIGHT.
STRAIN AND SWEETEN TO TASTE.

MUSCLE CRAMPS

MUSCLE CRAMPS DURING PREGNANCY CAN OCCUR DUE TO CHANGES IN CIRCULATION, INCREASED WEIGHT, AND THE STRAIN ON MUSCLES AND LIGAMENTS, AS WELL AS POTENTIAL DEFICIENCIES IN ESSENTIAL NUTRIENTS LIKE CALCIUM AND MAGNESIUM.

HERBS/REMEDIES: MAGNESIUM SUPPLEMENTS, BANANAS, WARM COMPRESSES

CRAMP EASE TEA:
1 PART SKULLCAP
1 PART NETTLE
½ PART CRAMP BARK
¼ PART TURMERIC
¼ PART GINGER

ADD CRAMP BARK, GINGER, AND TURMERIC TO 1 CUP OF WATER.
ADD TO COLD WATER AND BRING TO A SIMMER OVER LOW HEAT FOR 15 MINUTES
REMOVE FROM HEAT AND ADD SKULLCAP AND NETTLE LEAVES TO THE HOT WATER AND LET STEEP FOR 10 MINUTES COVERED. STRAIN, SWEETEN AS DESIRED.

Why Bitter Is Essential

Bitterness is often an overlooked and underappreciated taste in modern diets, yet it holds significant importance in maintaining overall health and well-being. In many traditional diets around the world, bitter foods and herbs have long been recognized for their medicinal properties and their ability to stimulate digestion, support liver function, and balance the body's internal systems. Bitter foods activate receptors on the tongue that send signals to the brain, stimulating the production of digestive enzymes and bile. This process not only aids in breaking down food more efficiently but also helps in the absorption of nutrients. Additionally, the stimulation of bile production by bitter compounds supports the liver's detoxification processes, which is crucial for maintaining overall health. Regular consumption of bitter foods can help regulate appetite, reduce sugar cravings, and promote a sense of balance in the digestive system. During pregnancy, many women experience this condition and bitter foods and herbs can play a supportive role in alleviating morning sickness. The bitter taste stimulates digestive secretions, which can help settle the stomach and reduce nausea.

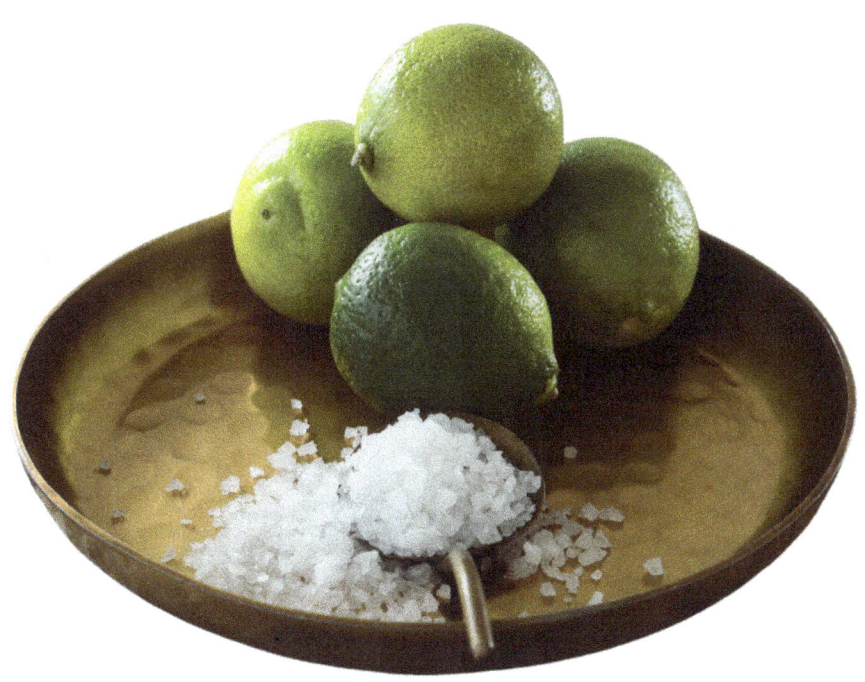

Herbs for Cough & Cold Support in Pregnancy

ECHINACEA
Echinacea purpurea / angustifolia

ECHINACEA IS TAKEN YEAR ROUND BY MANY AS AN IMMUNE SYSTEM TONIC. IT IS BEST TO USE THIS HERB IN ISOLATED INSTANCES. THIS HERB IS BEST USED AGAINST MICROBIAL INFECTIONS DUE TO ITS EFFECTIVENESS AGAINST BACTERIA & VIRUSES. IT IS ALSO GREAT TO USE EXTERNALLY AS WELL.

ELDERFLOWER
Sambucus nigra

THIS FLOWER IS BEST KNOWN FOR ITS POSITIVE EFFECTS DURING COLD & FLU SEASON. ELDERFLOWERS ARE AN IMMUNE BOOSTER THAT CAN TURN AROUND COLD SYMPTOMS AS WELL AS CLEAR CATARRH IN THE SINUSES AND UPPER RESPIRATORY TRACT.

ELECAMPANE
Inula helenium

THIS ROOT IS COMMONLY USED FOR ITS CAPABILITY TO RELIEVE MUCUS CONDITIONS ASSOCIATED WITH THE LUNGS. TYPICALLY ELECAMPANE IS USED WITH OTHER HERBS GOOD FOR COLDS AND CONGESTIONS.

ELEUTHERO
Eleutherococcus senticosus

THIS ROOT IS VERY EFFECTIVE IN BOOSTING THE IMMUNE SYSTEM AND HELPS TO SUPPORT ADRENAL HEALTH. IT IS A MEMBER OF THE GINSENG FAMILY AND BEST WHEN USED AS AN ADAPTOGEN INCREASING STAMINA AND ENERGY.

GINGER
Zingiber officinale

USED AS A DIAPHORETIC IN BREAKING A FEVER. THIS HERB IS ANTIVIRAL AND HELPS WITH ALLERGIES, ASTHMA, AND CHOLESTEROL. GINGER ALSO INCREASES CIRCULATION, WARMS THE WOMB, AND IS USED AS A UTERINE CLEANSER.

MARSHMALLOW RT
Althaea officinalis

THE HIGH MUCILAGINOUS CONTENT OF MARSHMALLOW ROOT MAKES IT A USEFUL REMEDY FOR COUGHS AND COLDS. IT IS ESPECIALLY EFFECTIVE IN RELIEVING COUGHS DUE TO COLDS, BRONCHITIS, OR RESPIRATORY TRACT DISEASES WITH FORMATION OF MUCUS.

MULLEIN
Verbascum thapsus

WHEN TAKEN INTERNALLY THIS HERB IS EFFECTIVE AT BREAKING UP CONGESTION AND SOOTHING THE MUCUS MEMBRANES IN THE CHEST. IT IS OFTEN USED WHEN THERE IS A PAINFUL, NON-PRODUCTIVE COUGH.

PLANTAIN
Plantago major

THIS HERB IS GREAT TO USE FOR SOOTHING AND HELPING TO REDUCE CONGESTION. THE LEAVES ARE GOOD FOR DRAWING OUT SPLINTERS AND LOCALIZED INFLAMMATION FROM THE BODY. PLANTAIN IS HIGHLY NUTRITIVE, A UTERINE TONIC, A LAXATIVE, AN ANTI-INFLAMMATORY AND CAN BE ADDED TO EVERYDAY FOODS.

SPEARMINT
Mentha spicata

THIS HERB IS EFFECTIVE IN ASSISTING THE BODY IN TOXIN REMOVAL. SPEARMINT IS ALSO HELPFUL FOR OPENING CONGESTED AIRWAYS WHICH IN TURN HELP TO IMPROVE BREATHING.

Recipe for Pregnancy Cold & Cough Tea

INGREDIENTS

½ CUP DRIED ROSEHIPS
½ CUP ELDERBERRIES
¼ CUP DRIED ELDER FLOWERS
¼ CUP DRIED ECHINACEA HERB (ECHINACEA SPP.)
2 TBL DRIED ORANGE RIND
2 TBL DRIED MULLIEN LEAF
1 TBL DRIED GINGER / 2" OF RAW GINGER SLICED
2 TBL DRIED SPEARMINT LEAF

INSTRUCTIONS

Stir all dry ingredients together in a medium-sized bowl until well-mixed, then store in an airtight container for up to 1 year.

To steep, add elderberries and echinacea to the water. If using raw ginger, add it to the pot. Bring to a boil then reduce heat and simmer for 7-10 minutes, then bring it back to a boil and remove from heat.

Add the remaining tea mixture to the boiled water, cover, and steep for 10-15 minutes.

Strain out the herbs and enjoy.

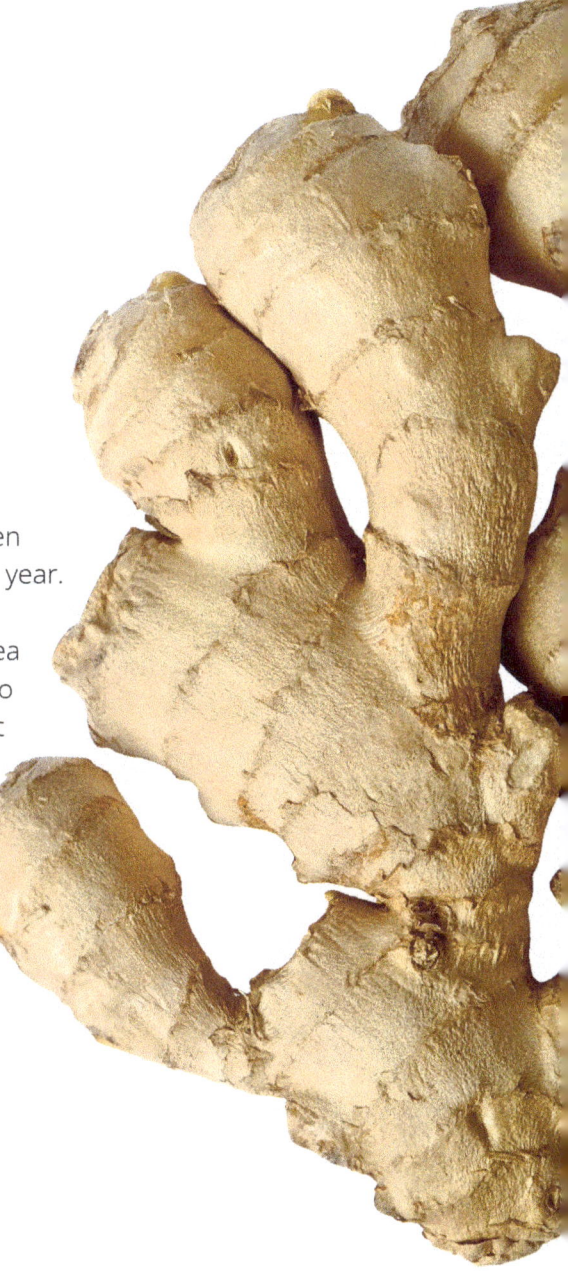

TINCTURE

THIS TINCTURE HAS IMMUNE SUPPORTIVE AND WARMING HERBS. YOU CAN USE AS A BASE AND ADD OTHER HERBS LIKE MULLEIN AND ELDERBERRY

COOTIE TINCTURE
1 PART ELEUTHERO
1 PART ECHINACEA
½ PART GINGER ROOT
½ PART LEMON BALM

TAKE 1-3 TIMES A DAY AT THE ONSET OF COLD OR FLU SYMPTOMS.
YOU CAN MIX THE TINCTURE INTO A SMALL AMOUNT OF WARM WATER OR HERBAL TEA.
*SEE TINCTURE INSTRUCTIONS IN HERBAL PREPARATIONS

STEAM

A HERBAL STEAM HELPS OPEN NASAL PASSAGES, CLEAR SINUSES, AND SOOTHE RESPIRATORY DISCOMFORT WHILE PROVIDING CALMING AND ANTI-INFLAMMATORY BENEFITS, MAKING IT A GENTLE AND EFFECTIVE REMEDY FOR COLD AND FLU SYMPTOMS DURING PREGNANCY.

1 PART PEPPERMINT
1 PART EUCALYPTUS
½ PART CHAMOMILE
½ PART LAVENDER

ADD A HANDFUL OF HERBS TO A BOWL OF HOT (NOT BOILING) WATER, THE STEAM SHOULD FEEL LIKE A WARM BATH. COVER YOUR HEAD WITH A TOWEL, AND INHALE THE STEAM FOR 5-10 MINUTES TO HELP CLEAR NASAL CONGESTION.

RUBIFACIENT SALVE

AN HERBAL RUBEFACIENT RUB INCREASES BLOOD FLOW TO THE APPLIED AREA, CREATING A WARMING SENSATION THAT HELPS RELIEVE MUSCLE TENSION, REDUCE PAIN, AND EASE COLDS AND CONGESTION BY PROMOTING THE RELEASE OF MUCUS AND OPENING AIRWAYS.

½ CUP CARRIER OIL (SUCH AS SWEET ALMOND OIL, JOJOBA OIL, OR COCONUT OIL)
10 DROPS OF GINGER ESSENTIAL OIL
8 DROPS OF EUCALYPTUS ESSENTIAL OIL
5 DROPS OF LAVENDER ESSENTIAL OIL
5 DROPS OF PEPPERMINT ESSENTIAL OIL USE SPARINGLY AND AVOID DIRECT CONTACT WITH THE FACE
1 TABLESPOON BEESWAX (OPTIONAL FOR A THICKER CONSISTENCY)

PREPARE THE BASE:
IF YOU PREFER A THICKER RUB, MELT THE BEESWAX IN A DOUBLE BOILER OVER LOW HEAT. ONCE MELTED, ADD THE CARRIER OIL AND STIR UNTIL WELL COMBINED. IF YOU PREFER A LIQUID RUB, SKIP THE BEESWAX AND DIRECTLY POUR THE CARRIER OIL INTO A GLASS BOWL.

ADD ESSENTIAL OILS:
REMOVE FROM HEAT AND LET IT COOL SLIGHTLY. ADD THE ESSENTIAL OILS (GINGER, EUCALYPTUS, LAVENDER, AND PEPPERMINT). STIR GENTLY TO COMBINE. THE QUALITY OF YOUR OILS MATTER. MAKE SURE YOU ARE USING QUALITY ESSENTIAL NOT FRAGRANCE OILS.

COOL AND STORE: POUR THE MIXTURE INTO A CLEAN, DARK GLASS JAR. LET IT COOL COMPLETELY BEFORE CLOSING THE LID. STORE IN A COOL, DARK PLACE.

APPLICATION: APPLY A SMALL AMOUNT OF THE RUB TO THE CHEST, BACK, OR FEET TO HELP RELIEVE CONGESTION AND PROVIDE A WARMING SENSATION. YOU CAN USE IT 2-3 TIMES A DAY AS NEEDED.

Botanical Support
FOR COMPLEX PREGNANCY COMPLAINTS

SPOTTING

1. RED RASPBERRY LEAF (RUBUS IDAEUS)
    - DESCRIPTION: STRENGTHENS AND TONES UTERINE MUSCLES, SUPPORTING A HEALTHIER UTERINE ENVIRONMENT.
    - USE: CONSUMED AS TEA OR INFUSION. SAFE THROUGHOUT PREGNANCY.
    - RECOMMENDATION: START MODERATELY IN EARLY PREGNANCY (8 OZ OF TEA A DAY) AND INCREASE IN THE SECOND AND THIRD TRIMESTERS.
2. CRAMP BARK (VIBURNUM OPULUS)
    - DESCRIPTION: ANTISPASMODIC; RELAXES UTERINE MUSCLES AND REDUCES CRAMPING.
    - USE: TINCTURE OR TEA. RECOMMENDED FOR MILD UTERINE CRAMPING AND SPOTTING.
    - RECOMMENDATION: SAFE DURING PREGNANCY WITH HEALTHCARE GUIDANCE.
3. BLACK HAW (VIBURNUM PRUNIFOLIUM)
    - DESCRIPTION: RELAXES THE UTERUS, REDUCES CRAMPS, MAY PREVENT MISCARRIAGE.
    - USE: TINCTURE OR TEA FOR UTERINE RELAXATION AND SPOTTING.
4. PARTRIDGE BERRY (MITCHELLA REPENS)
    - DESCRIPTION: UTERINE-TONING PROPERTIES, PREVENTS MISCARRIAGE, SUPPORTS PREGNANCY.
    - USE: TINCTURE OR PART OF AN HERBAL FORMULA.
    - RECOMMENDATION: USED IN SECOND AND THIRD TRIMESTERS FOR UTERINE SUPPORT.
5. NETTLE (URTICA DIOICA)
    - DESCRIPTION: NUTRITIVE HERB, RICH IN IRON AND CALCIUM, STRENGTHENS THE UTERUS.
    - USE: INFUSION OR TEA, SAFE THROUGHOUT PREGNANCY.
    - RECOMMENDATION: USE AS A DAILY TONIC.
6. WILD YAM (DIOSCOREA VILLOSA)
    - DESCRIPTION: ANTISPASMODIC, REDUCES UTERINE DISCOMFORT.
    - USE: TYPICALLY IN TINCTURE FORM TO PREVENT MISCARRIAGE AND REDUCE SPOTTING.

GESTATIONAL DIABETES

1. CINNAMON (CINNAMOMUM VERUM)
    - DESCRIPTION: IMPROVES INSULIN SENSITIVITY, REGULATES BLOOD SUGAR.
    - USE: ADDED TO FOODS, TEAS, OR AS A SUPPLEMENT.
2. NETTLE (URTICA DIOICA)
    - DESCRIPTION: RICH IN MAGNESIUM, SUPPORTS BLOOD SUGAR REGULATION.
    - USE: TEA OR INFUSION, SAFE DURING PREGNANCY.
3. DANDELION ROOT (TARAXACUM OFFICINALE)
    - DESCRIPTION: LIVER SUPPORT, IMPROVES GLUCOSE METABOLISM.
    - USE: TEA, TINCTURE, OR POWDERED FORM.
4. GINGER (ZINGIBER OFFICINALE)
    - DESCRIPTION: ANTI-INFLAMMATORY, IMPROVES INSULIN SENSITIVITY.
    - USE: TEA, FRESH IN FOOD, OR SUPPLEMENTS.

PRE-ECLAMSPIA

1. NETTLE (URTICA DIOICA)
   - DESCRIPTION: RICH IN MINERALS, DIURETIC, REDUCES FLUID RETENTION.
   - USE: TEA OR INFUSION, SAFE DURING PREGNANCY.
2. DANDELION LEAF (TARAXACUM OFFICINALE)
   - DESCRIPTION: NUTRITIVE, DIURETIC, REDUCES SWELLING, LOWERS BLOOD PRESSURE.
   - USE: TEA OR FRESH IN SALADS.
3. HAWTHORN (CRATAEGUS SPP.)
   - DESCRIPTION: SUPPORTS CARDIOVASCULAR FUNCTION, REGULATES BLOOD PRESSURE.
   - USE: TEA OR TINCTURE, BEST USED UNDER PROFESSIONAL GUIDANCE.
4. GARLIC (ALLIUM SATIVUM)
   - DESCRIPTION: CARDIOVASCULAR BENEFITS, LOWERS BLOOD PRESSURE.
   - USE: FRESH OR IN SUPPLEMENTS.
5. CHAMOMILE (MATRICARIA CHAMOMILLA)
   - DESCRIPTION: CALMING, REDUCES STRESS, MILD DIURETIC.
   - USE: TEA, SAFE DURING PREGNANCY.
6. LEMON BALM (MELISSA OFFICINALIS)
   - DESCRIPTION: CALMING, MILDLY HYPOTENSIVE.
   - USE: TEA OR TINCTURE, SAFE IN MODERATE AMOUNTS.

LOW PLATELETS

1. NETTLE (URTICA DIOICA)
   - DESCRIPTION: NUTRITIVE, BLOOD-BUILDING, INCREASES PLATELET COUNT.
   - USE: TEA, TINCTURE, INFUSION. SAFE DURING PREGNANCY.
2. ALFALFA (MEDICAGO SATIVA)
   - DESCRIPTION: NUTRIENT-DENSE, RICH IN VITAMIN K, SUPPORTS PLATELET FUNCTION.
   - USE: TEA, CAPSULES, SMOOTHIES. SAFE IN DIETARY AMOUNTS DURING PREGNANCY.
3. RED RASPBERRY LEAF (RUBUS IDAEUS)
   - DESCRIPTION: RICH IN NUTRIENTS, SUPPORTS OVERALL BLOOD HEALTH.
   - USE: COMMONLY AS TEA, SAFE IN MODERATION, ESPECIALLY IN EARLY PREGNANCY.
4. ASTRAGALUS (ASTRAGALUS MEMBRANACEUS)
   - DESCRIPTION: ADAPTOGENIC, BOOSTS IMMUNITY, SUPPORTS BLOOD HEALTH.
   - USE: DECOCTION, TINCTURE, SUPPLEMENT.
5. DANDELION LEAF (TARAXACUM OFFICINALE)
   - DESCRIPTION: RICH IN VITAMINS, SUPPORTS BLOOD CLOTTING AND HEALTH.
   - USE: TEA, FRESH IN SALADS, TINCTURE.
6. DONG QUAI (ANGELICA SINENSIS)
   - DESCRIPTION: SUPPORTS BLOOD HEALTH AND CIRCULATION.
   - USE: TYPICALLY IN COMBINATION WITH OTHER HERBS.
7. PAPAYA LEAVES (CARICA PAPAYA)
   - DESCRIPTION: TRADITIONALLY SUPPORTS PLATELET PRODUCTION.
   - USE: EXTRACT AS TEA, JUICE, OR FRESH LEAVES IN REMEDIES.

"Labor is a sacred ceremony, a rite of passage that connects us with the wisdom of our ancestors and the spirit of the earth."
-Elisabeth (Libby) Davis
Cherokee Traditional Midwife

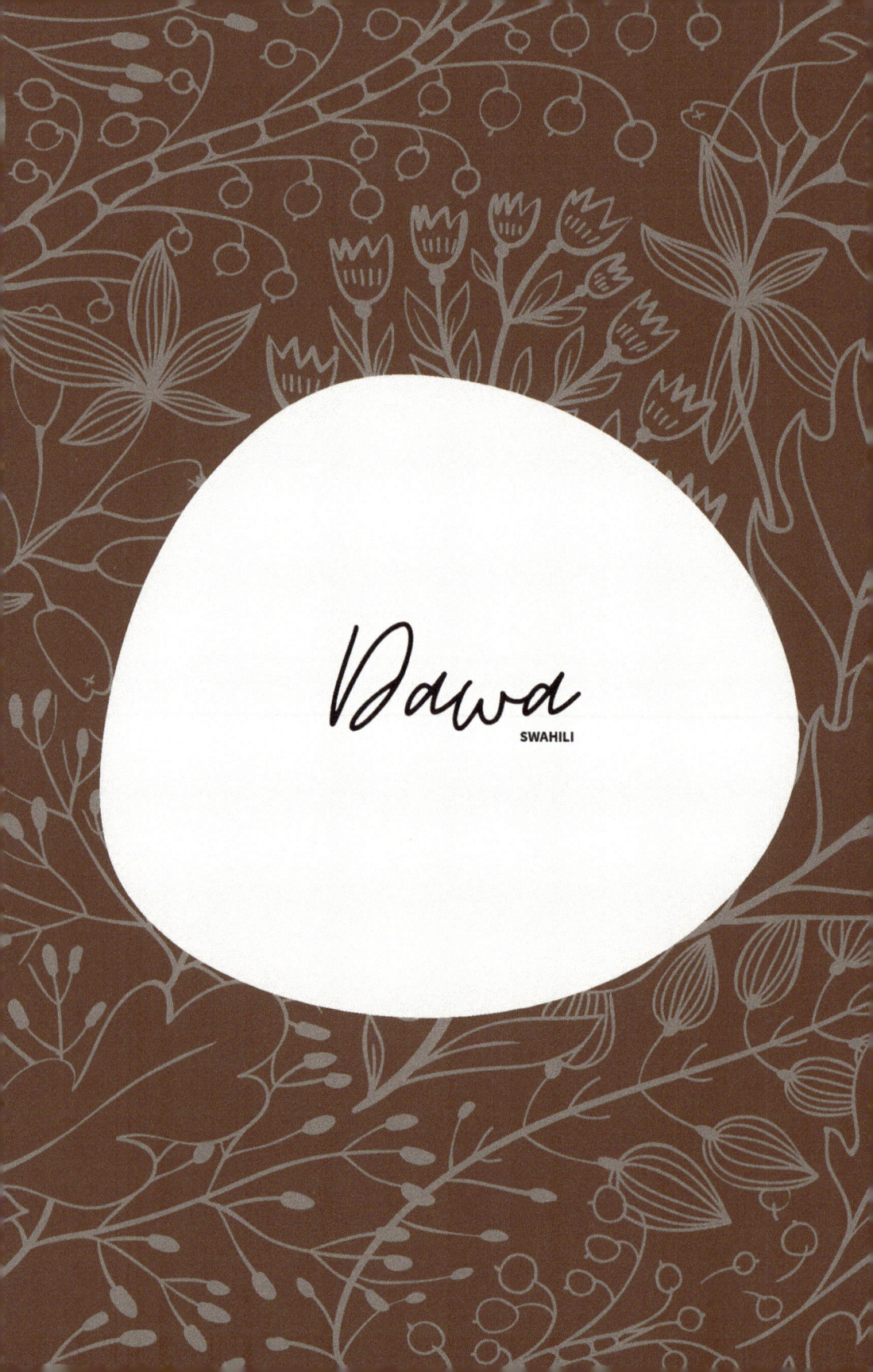

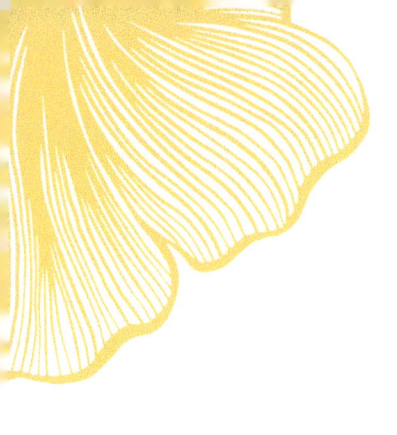

chapter 5

Innate Wisdom of The Body
Botanical Support for Labor
Miscarriage
Go Get The Spirit

"Labor is a time of transformation and deep inner strength. Herbs can support the body in its journey, but the real magic comes from within the birthing person, who is both the creator and the guide."

Rosemary Gladstar
Herbalist and Author

The Sacred Innate Wisdom of a Woman's Body

The process of labor stands as one of the most profound expressions of a woman's innate wisdom. Within her, the sacred blueprint of birth is etched deep into her being—a testament to the timeless connection between body, spirit, and the cycles of nature.

A woman's body is designed to bring forth new life with remarkable intelligence. From the moment labor begins, the body awakens to a rhythm that is ancient and primal. Each contraction is a powerful dance of muscle and will that guides the baby gently toward the world.

This sacred wisdom is an inherent part of the birthing experience. The body knows precisely how to navigate this journey, drawing upon generations of ancestral knowledge and biological instinct. It is a process that transcends mere mechanics; it is a profound and sacred ritual, connecting the birthing person with the rhythms of the Earth and the lineage of women who have birthed before.

Herbs, in this context, play a supporting, not mandatory, role. They are companions offering comfort and enhancing the natural process, helping to smooth transitions and support the body's incredible journey with additional layers of care. They can help alleviate discomfort, support relaxation, and bolster strength, but their purpose is to honor and enhance the already innate birthing process and be of assistance if needed. The true magic of birth lies within the woman herself.

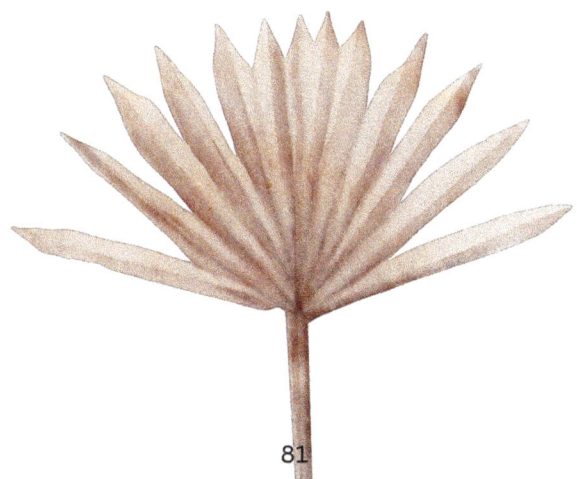

Botanical Support For Labor

HERBS TO FACILITATE LABOR

RED RASPBERRY LEAF Rubus idaeus	How to Use: Taken as a tea or in capsule form; traditionally consumed in the weeks leading up to labor to tone the uterus and during labor to facilitate contractions. Dangers: Generally considered safe, but high doses can cause excessive contractions; should be used with caution in the first trimester.
BLUE COHOSH Caulophyllum thalictroides	How to Use: Tincture or decoction taken to stimulate uterine contractions. Dangers: Should be used under supervision due to potential side effects such as nausea, increased blood pressure, and potential toxicity to the fetus if used improperly.
BLACK COHOSH Actaea racemosa	How to Use: Tincture or tea used to stimulate contractions and facilitate labor. Dangers: Can cause nausea, headache, and dizziness; should not be used early in pregnancy due to risk of miscarriage.
EVENING PRIMROSE OIL Oenothera biennis	How to Use: Taken orally or applied vaginally in the last weeks of pregnancy to soften the cervix. Dangers: Should not be used in early pregnancy; may cause mild gastrointestinal upset.
COTTON ROOT BARK Gossypium herbaceum	How to Use: Tincture or decoction used to stimulate uterine contractions and facilitate labor. Dangers: Should be used under supervision; can cause intense uterine contractions and should not be used in early pregnancy.
CLARY SAGE Salvia sclarea	How to Use: Used as an essential oil in aromatherapy to stimulate contractions and reduce anxiety. Dangers: Should be used with caution and not ingested; avoid use in early pregnancy.
CASTOR BEAN OIL Ricinus communis	Castor oil is a well-known natural remedy for inducing labor, typically taken orally in small amounts and often mixed with juice or another liquid to mask its taste. It works by stimulating the bowels, which can in turn trigger uterine contractions. It is often used when a mother is past her due date, but it should always be under the guidance of a midwife or healthcare provider as its efficacy and safety vary. Castor oil can cause very intense and painful contractions that might not lead to productive labor, along with side effects such as diarrhea, dehydration, nausea, and vomiting. Importantly, castor oil should never be used before the baby is full term, as it can induce premature labor. Some studies suggest it may be effective for certain individuals, while others show limited impact.

HERBS TO STABILIZE BLOOD PRESSURE DURING LABOR

HAWTHORNE BERRY Crataegus spp.	How to Use: Taken as a tea or tincture to support cardiovascular health and stabilize blood pressure. Dangers: Generally safe but should be used with caution in combination with other medications for heart conditions.
BLACK COHOSH Actaea racemosa	How to Use: Tincture or tea to help manage blood pressure and ease labor. Dangers: Can cause nausea, headache, and dizziness; should not be used early in pregnancy due to risk of miscarriage.
BLACK HAW Viburnum prunifolium	How to Use: Tincture: Taken in small doses, diluted in water. Decoction: Boil the root in water and consume. Medicinal Benefits: May Prevent Premature Labor: Relaxes the uterus and reduces contractions. Eases Labor Pains: Reduces muscle spasms and cramping. Stabilizes Blood Pressure: Helps maintain stable blood pressure during labor. Allergic Reactions: Possible skin rashes or gastrointestinal discomfort. Dangers: Not for long-term use due to potential adverse effects on liver and kidneys. Medication Interactions: May interact with blood pressure medications and anticoagulants; consult a healthcare provider before use.
LINDEN FLOWERS Tilia cordata	How to Use: Taken as a tea to calm nerves and stabilize blood pressure. Dangers: Generally safe; overuse can cause drowsiness.
SQUAW VINE* Mitchella repens	How to Use: Taken as a tea or tincture to support labor and stabilize blood pressure. Dangers: Should be used under supervision; not recommended for use in early pregnancy. *Also referred to as Partridgeberry in this book
SHEPHERD'S PURSE Capsella bursa-pastoris	How to Use: Tincture or infusion to stabilize blood pressure and control bleeding. Dangers: Should not be used during pregnancy due to its uterine-stimulating properties

HERBS FOR HEAVY BLEEDING

YARROW
Achillea millefolium

How to Use: Taken as a tea or tincture to control bleeding. Can also be used topically as a styptic. should not be used during pregnancy
Dangers: Generally considered safe when used appropriately. Use with caution if you are taking blood thinners. It may Interact with medications like sedatives, blood pressure medications, or drugs that affect blood clotting.

SHEPHERD'S PURSE
Capsella bursa-pastoris

How to Use: Tincture or infusion to reduce postpartum bleeding.
Dangers: Generally safe; should not be used during pregnancy due to its uterine-stimulating properties.

WITCH HAZEL
Hamamelis virginiana

How to Use: Tincture or external application to reduce bleeding and swelling.
Dangers: Generally safe for external use; internal use should be supervised due to potential liver toxicity.

YUNNAN BAIYO
Proprietary blend including Panax Notoginseng

How to Use: Traditionally used as a powder placed in a capsule to control heavy bleeding. Can be used as a vaginal suppository.
Dangers: Generally safe

Midwives and obstetricians caution that if you are soaking more than two sanitary pads in 30 minutes that you seek medical attention. Any fever, large clotting, or foul odor are signs of retained placenta and possible infection.

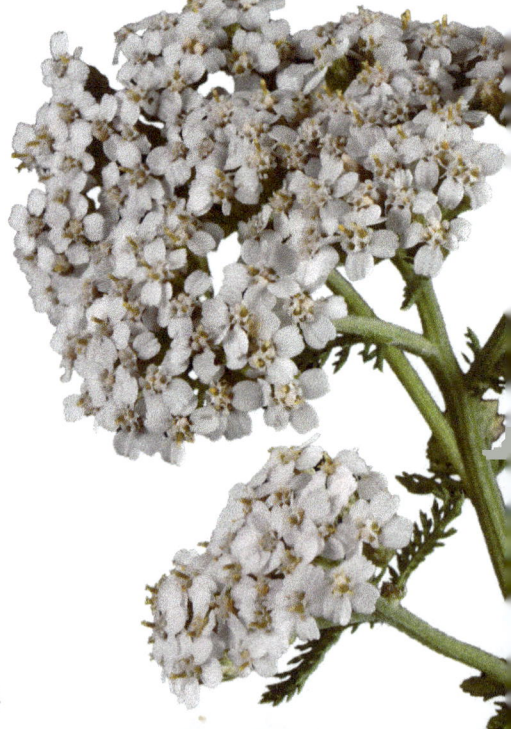

Reducing Postpartum Hemorrhage: The Role of Herbs and Oxytocin

Postpartum hemorrhage (PPH), defined as blood loss of 500 mL or more following vaginal delivery, remains one of the leading causes of maternal mortality worldwide, contributing to 25% of maternal deaths annually. Early PPH, occurring within the first 24 hours postpartum, accounts for most fatalities, while late PPH can occur between 24 hours and 12 weeks postpartum. Affecting 3%–8% of births, PPH is most often caused by uterine atony, responsible for approximately 70% of cases. Without timely intervention, PPH can lead to severe complications, including iron deficiency anemia, Sheehan's syndrome, impaired lactation, shock, and even death. In recent years, research has highlighted the potential of combining herbal remedies with pharmacological treatments like oxytocin to improve outcomes in managing PPH. A study involving 100 women at Shahid Sadoughi Hospital tested sublingual hydroalcoholic extract of Capsella bursa-pastoris (shepherd's purse) in combination with oxytocin. Results revealed significantly reduced postpartum bleeding in the group receiving the herbal extract alongside oxytocin compared to the control group, with only mild side effects reported. Similarly, a trial involving 120 women assessed the effects of grape seed powder in doses of 50–150 mg, combined with oxytocin, on postpartum bleeding. Findings demonstrated a notable reduction in blood loss among all grape seed powder groups compared to those receiving oxytocin alone, underscoring the efficacy of this integrative approach.

Standalone herbal remedies also show promise as alternatives to synthetic drugs, particularly in settings where access to conventional treatments is limited. Dill (Anethum graveolens) extract has been shown to significantly reduce postpartum bleeding, with one study reporting average blood loss of 52.6 ± 23.2 mL in the dill group compared to 87.6 ± 40.4 mL in the oxytocin group. Similarly, Phoenix dactylifera (dates) have demonstrated effectiveness in reducing postpartum bleeding. In one study, 62 women receiving 50 g of dates after placental removal experienced better outcomes than those given 10 units of oxytocin. Another study with 90 women found that consuming 100 g of dates daily reduced bleeding from day 2 to day 10 postpartum, although the overall duration of bleeding remained unchanged.

Conventional treatments for PPH include mechanical, pharmacological, and surgical methods. Pharmacological options, such as oxytocin, Ergomethrin, Syntocinone, Carboprost, and Misoprostol, are commonly used to stimulate uterine contractions and prevent uterine atony. Mechanical interventions, such as bladder drainage and bimanual uterine compression massage, and surgical options, such as uterine artery ligation, are also employed in severe cases where other methods fail.

Given growing concerns about chemical exposure, particularly during breastfeeding, the integration of herbal remedies with pharmacological treatments offers a promising path forward. Compounds found in herbs, such as flavonoids, tannins, omega-6 fatty acids, and vitamins C and E, may play a critical role in controlling bleeding while reducing dependency on synthetic drugs. Studies suggest that this collaborative approach not only enhances maternal health outcomes but also minimizes risks associated with chemical medications, providing safer alternatives for mothers and their infants.

In conclusion, the integration of herbal remedies and oxytocin represents an innovative and effective approach to managing postpartum hemorrhage. By combining traditional knowledge with modern medical practices, this strategy aligns with the evolving landscape of postpartum care, offering a holistic, safe, and efficient means to support maternal health. Ongoing research into these collaborative methods will further refine and advance maternal healthcare practices, ensuring better outcomes for women worldwide.

See reference section at end of book for full study info (Khojastehfard et al. 62)

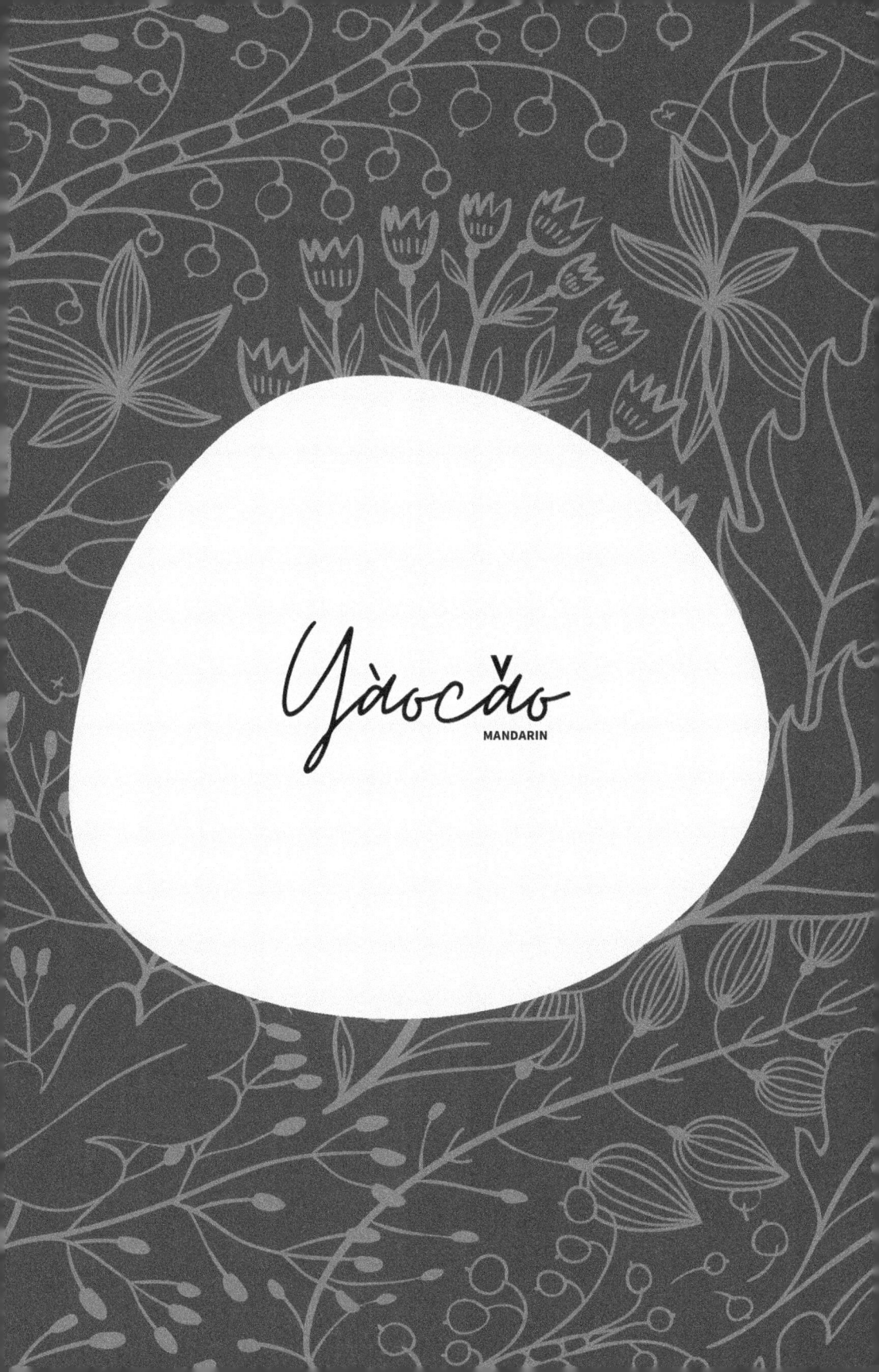

A Note On Blue Cohosh

Blue cohosh, also known as Pappoose Root or Squawroot, grows throughout North America. Blue cohosh (Caulophyllum thalictroides) is not in the same family as black cohosh (Cimicifuga racemosa). It is often assumed that they are related and they are both used to support female health concerns. Blue Cohosh has been used by birth workers in North America since time in memoriam. It is believed that it functions similar to the hormone estrogen. It has been used to stimulate the uterus and bring labor. Also to ease cramps, muscle spasms, inflammation of the uterus and overgrowth of uterine tissue (endometriosis). Although it has been used traditionally for some time, it is now considered controversial to utilize blue cohosh to start labor. There is in vitro evidence that blue cohosh may have embryo toxic and tetragenic properties.

These chemicals can be toxic to the mother, can cause birth defects when ingested in early pregnancy, and can cause severe heart problems in the newborn when taken late in pregnancy. It may disrupt the mitochondrial function and narrow vessels that carry blood to the heart which can decrease cardiac oxygen levels. There have been reported cases of perinatal stroke, acute myocardial infarction, multi organ hypoxic injury, and permanent central nervous system damage.   In full transparency, there were questionable variables in some of the case studies where these incidents were reported. For example, the birthing person taking more than the midwife's recommended dose, another with the birthing person having ingested a blend of herbs containing blue and black cohosh in unknown amounts, and another incident where the tincture was tested but the tests failed to provide conclusive results.

If blue cohosh is used to facilitate labor, it should be administered by a midwife or OB/GYN. However, if you choose to use it, it is encouraged that you use the smallest amount possible for the shortest amount of time needed, and that the birthing person and child are closely monitored.

Motherwort: Leonurus cardiaca

Motherwort (Leonurus cardiaca) is valued for its calming and grounding properties. It has been used for centuries to assist women through various stages of motherhood, particularly during labor and postpartum.

Calming and Grounding Effects: Motherwort has the ability to calm the nervous system and is often used to alleviate anxiety, stress, and nervous tension, which can be particularly beneficial during labor. Its grounding effect can anchor a mother in the present moment, helping her to remain centered and focused during the intense experience of childbirth. Midwife TBAMJIK, for example, likes to drop some motherwort tincture on her clients' tongues after they have been laboring, just before it's time to push. This practice can help the mother stay calm and present, easing the transition to the final stages of childbirth.

Support During Labor: Motherwort's antispasmodic properties help to relax smooth muscles, making it useful for reducing uterine cramping and spasms during labor.

Heart Tonic: As a heart tonic, motherwort supports cardiovascular health by helping to regulate blood pressure and heart rate. This is particularly important during labor when the body is under significant physical stress. By promoting a healthy heart function, motherwort can contribute to a safer and smoother birthing process.

Postpartum Support: Motherwort is also beneficial postpartum. It helps to ease afterpains, reduce anxiety, and support emotional balance. Its mildly sedative properties can help new mothers get the rest they need, promoting overall recovery and well-being.

How to Use Motherwort
Tincture: Fresh motherwort tincture is the most common form used in herbalism. It can be taken in small doses, usually diluted in water. During labor, a few drops under the tongue can provide quick relief from anxiety and help manage labor pains.

Infusion: An infusion of dried motherwort leaves in hot water can be sipped throughout the day for postpartum support, aiding emotional balance and uterine health. While generally safe, it may interact with medications for heart or blood pressure.

"Grief in our traditions is not just about tears; it is about the acknowledgment of life and spirit, of the connection that was and the connection that remains. Miscarriage is part of that cycle, a moment where the spirit moves on, but love stays behind."

Paula Gunn Allen
(Laguna Pueblo-Sioux, Poet, and Scholar)

MISCARRIAGE

Many cultures often view miscarriage through a lens of spiritual and communal understanding, recognizing it as a natural part of life and a significant event for the woman and her family. The beliefs surrounding miscarriage vary among different Indigenous groups, but many share a common reverence for the life that was lost and the woman's experience.

In many Indigenous traditions, miscarriage is seen as a moment where the spirit of the child chose not to stay, and this decision is respected and honored. The spirit is often believed to be on a journey, perhaps needing more time before entering the physical world. This perspective can bring comfort to the grieving family, as it frames the loss within a spiritual context rather than viewing it as a failure or tragedy.

Support for the family, especially the woman, is deeply rooted in community practices. Elders, midwives, and healers often play key roles in offering emotional and spiritual guidance. Ceremonies or rituals may be conducted to honor the lost spirit, cleanse the woman, and help her heal emotionally and physically. Herbal remedies are commonly used to support the woman's body in recovering, soothe her spirit, and prepare her for future pregnancies if she so desires.

The family is enveloped in care, with the community coming together to provide meals, share stories, and offer their presence. In many cultures, it is believed that the woman should be surrounded by love and support to help her grieve and find peace. The acknowledgment of the miscarriage as a shared experience rather than a solitary burden helps the family heal together, reaffirming their connection to each other and their ancestors.

This holistic approach ensures that the loss is honored, the woman's wellbeing is prioritized, and the family is supported both emotionally and spiritually.

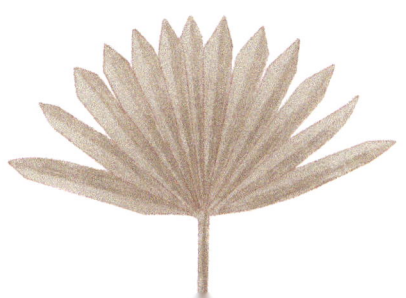

Botanical Support Miscarriage

BLUE VERVAIN
Verbena hastata

Known for its calming and relaxing properties. It can be used to help soothe emotional distress and promote a sense of peace during the healing process after a miscarriage. Additionally, Blue Vervain has been traditionally used to support the female reproductive system and may aid in toning and balancing the uterus.

BLACK HAW
Viburnum prunifolium
CRAMP BARK
Viburnum opulus

Used separately or together, these herbs help ease uterine cramping and muscle tension, providing relief from physical discomfort during and after a miscarriage.

MOTHERWORT
Leonurus cardiaca

Calming the nervous system and easing emotional distress, providing comfort during the grieving process. It also supports the uterus, helping to gently tone and soothe it as the body heals.

NETTLE
Urtica dioica

Rich in iron and nutrients, it helps replenish the body after blood loss, supports overall vitality, and aids in recovery after a miscarriage.

PARTRIDGE BERRY
Mitchella repens

Traditionally used to regulate menstrual cycles and promote uterine health, it can support the uterus in returning to balance after a miscarriage.

RED RASPBERRY LEAF
Rubus idaeus

Strengthens and tones the uterus, helping to reduce bleeding and support the healing process after a miscarriage.

YARROW
Achillea millefolium

Helps to reduce excessive bleeding and promote circulation, supporting the body in managing blood flow during a miscarriage.

Additional Support For Loss

- Boosting Oxytocin: Engage in activities that naturally increase oxytocin, the "love hormone," such as hugging, slow dancing, cuddling with a loved one, or spending time with pets. These activities can help elevate mood and ease emotional pain.

- Ceremony or Ritual: Create a personal or cultural ceremony to honor the lost spirit, offering a sense of closure and spiritual healing. This can include lighting candles, writing a letter to the baby, or making an offering to the earth.

- Reaching Out for Support: Contact local pregnancy loss support groups, a therapist, or a trusted friend or family member to share your experience and receive emotional support.

- Rest and Self-Care: Prioritize rest and gentle self-care, including nourishing foods, warm baths, and quiet time. Listen to your body and give yourself permission to grieve and heal at your own pace.

- Womb Massage: Gentle abdominal massage can help soothe the uterus, promote healing, and connect you with your body. This can be done by a trained practitioner or with self-massage techniques.

You Have To Go Get The Spirit

In many Indigenous cultures, birth is seen as a sacred journey where the mother embarks on a spiritual voyage to the heavens to retrieve the soul of her baby. This belief reflects a deep connection between the earthly and spiritual realms, honoring the profound role of the mother as both a life-giver and a spiritual guide.

According to this tradition, the act of giving birth is not merely physical but a mystical experience. As labor begins, it is believed that the mother's soul rises from her body and ascends to the heavens. In this ethereal realm, she seeks out the spirit of her child, who is waiting to be brought into the world. The journey is one of courage and love, as the mother ventures into the unknown to find and bring back the soul that will join her family on Earth.

This story of birth is both beautiful and empowering. It portrays the mother as a powerful and spiritual being who bridges the gap between worlds. She is entrusted with the sacred task of guiding a new soul into existence; an act that honors her strength, wisdom, and deep connection to the divine. The baby's arrival is not seen as a mere biological event but as a reunion of spirits—a moment when the mother returns to her body, carrying with her the soul of her child, ready to welcome them into the world.

This belief also emphasizes the deep bond between mother and child as their souls are intertwined even before birth. The mother's journey to the heavens symbolizes the lengths to which she will go for her child, underscoring the love, dedication, and spiritual responsibility inherent in motherhood.

In telling this story of birth, Indigenous cultures offer a profound narrative that frames childbirth as a sacred and transformative experience. It is a reminder of the spiritual dimensions of life and the unique role of women as the bearers of new life, bridging the gap between the seen and unseen, the earthly and the divine. This perspective celebrates the miracle of birth not just as the beginning of a new life, but as the fulfillment of a divine journey, shared by mother and child, that continues long after their souls have returned to Earth.

"In the moment of birth, a mother journeys to the spiritual realm, drawing on the strength of the ancestors to guide the baby's soul into this world. It is a dance of love, life, and spirit, where two souls meet in the timeless space of creation."

Shafia Monroe
Traditional Midwife, Founder of the International Center for Traditional Childbearing

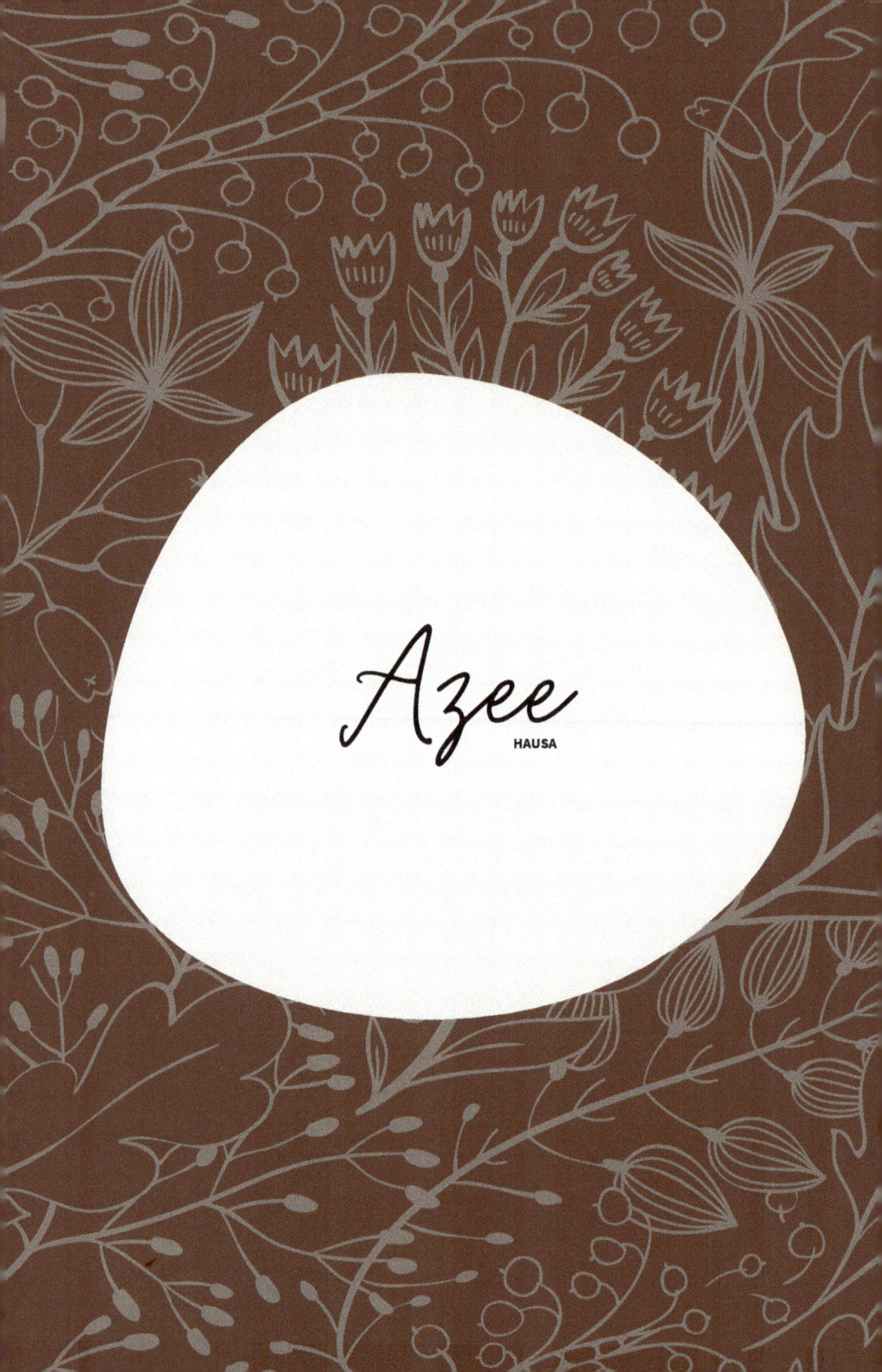

chapter 6

Tradition in Postpartum Care
Botanical Support For Postpartum
Postpartum Wellness Recipes

"Rather than limiting postpartum to an arbitrary 6 weeks, many midwives, childbirth educators, and postpartum doulas are encouraging women to see the postpartum as a fourth trimester, thus allowing themselves at least a full three months for physical recovery, spiritual integration, and emotional assimilation. Even three months, many experts agree, may be too short a time. Many mothers say it was closer to 8 months before they began to feel more settled in their role as mother, and able to regain a sense of personal identity and clarity."

Aviva Romm
Midwife, Herbalist, MD,

The Role of Herbs in Traditional Postpartum Care

Herbs have long been an integral part of traditional postpartum care across various cultures. They offer holistic support to new mothers, addressing physical recovery, emotional well-being, and overall nourishment during the postpartum period. This time, often referred to as the "fourth trimester," is crucial for a mother's healing and adjustment to new motherhood. Traditional herbal practices provide a wealth of knowledge and remedies that have been used for generations to support this transition.

Postpartum recovery involves more than just physical healing from childbirth; it also encompasses recuperation from the extensive changes and demands placed on a woman's body during pregnancy. Throughout the nine months of gestation, a mother's body undergoes significant physiological changes and nutrient depletion. Essential reserves, including calcium, iron, magnesium, and other vital nutrients, are drawn upon to support the growing fetus, leaving a new mother feeling exhausted and in urgent need of replenishment. Calcium, crucial for bone health and the proper functioning of muscles and nerves, is especially impacted as it is transferred to the baby for bone development. Similarly, iron levels can drop due to blood loss during delivery, making iron-rich herbs essential for restoring energy and preventing anemia. Magnesium, which supports muscle and nerve function and helps manage stress, also requires replenishment. Additionally, the body's overall vitamin and mineral reserves, including B vitamins and vitamin C, are often diminished after pregnancy and childbirth.

Traditional herbal practices address these needs by providing remedies that support physical recovery, emotional well-being, and overall nourishment during the postpartum period. Herbs are used to replenish depleted nutrients, support healing, and stabilize mood, playing a crucial role in helping new mothers regain their strength and balance. By integrating herbs into postpartum care through remedies and foods, women can benefit from centuries of wisdom that supports a holistic recovery, addressing both the physical and emotional aspects of this transformative period. Herbs can play a vital role in replenishing these essential nutrients, offering both herbal remedies and culinary options to support a new mother's recovery and well-being during the postpartum period.

A Global Perspective on Postpartum Care: Embracing Universal Wisdom

In examining postpartum care practices across diverse cultures, you will notice that all the aunties, sisters, mothers, and great-grandmothers are saying the same thing when it comes to postpartum recovery. Despite vast geographical distances and cultural differences, the common thread weaving through these approaches emphasizes warming, easily digestible foods, ample rest for at least a month, the use of herbs, and strong community support.

- Food: From Asia, Africa, to the Americas, new mothers are guided towards consuming nourishing, easily digestible foods. These foods are not merely about sustenance; they are believed to restore balance and vitality after the exhaustive demands of childbirth. For instance, in various Asian cultures, postpartum diets often center around nutrient-rich soups and stews made from bone broth and infused with restorative herbs. This not only assists in the transition to motherhood but also helps rejuvenate the body in preparation for menopause later in life. Many cultures understand the impact postpartum care can have on menopause.

- Rest: Rest is a universally emphasized aspect of postpartum care. Across cultures, there is a clear acknowledgment of the need for new mothers to pause and recover from the physical strains of labor. This can be challenging in opposition to the hustle culture and the lack of adequate maternal/paternal leave and support. Many traditions advocate for extended periods of bed rest, reduced activity, and a concentrated focus on bonding with the newborn. This common practice illustrates a collective awareness of the essential nature of rest for physical healing and emotional stability during the postpartum period.

- Botanical Support: Herbal remedies further highlight the global consensus on postpartum care. From the herbal teas of Eastern Europe to the traditional practices of Indigenous communities in North America, herbs are employed to support various aspects of postpartum recovery. Herbs used in many cultures assist in uterine recovery and nutrient replenishment. The widespread use of these natural remedies speaks to a shared wisdom about the benefits of herbs and their role in healing after childbirth.

- Social Support :Equally important is the role of social support in postpartum care. The presence of a supportive network is a universal aspect of postpartum traditions. This network provides practical help, emotional reassurance, and guidance based on traditional knowledge. The consistent emphasis on community support underscores a collective understanding of the nurturing environment needed for a new mother's recovery.

These commonalities across cultures highlight valuable traditional wisdom that deserves recognition. These practices have evolved from generations of knowledge. Embracing these time-honored approaches honors a global heritage and enhances support for new mothers.

"Culture may shift and evolve, but birth remains a universal truth—a shared human experience that deserves to be held with care, reverence, and respect. When we restore this balance, when we care for mothers in all their power and vulnerability, we care for the very essence of our future. Because if we do not care for the mothers, who will care for the rest of us?"

—Charlotte Brielle
Founder and Executive Director of Wombs of the World

Botanical Support FOR POSTPARTUM

AMARANTH
Amaranthus spp

AMARANTH LEAVES HELP REPLENISH VITAL NUTRIENTS LOST DURING PREGNANCY AND CHILDBIRTH ESPECIALLY IRON AND CALCIUM. IT SUPPORTS BLOOD PRODUCTION AND OVERALL VITALITY. THEY ARE TYPICALLY COOKED AS LEAFY GREENS, ADDED TO TEAS, SOUPS, OR USED IN STEWS TO BOOST NUTRITION.

ASHWAGANDA
Withania somnifera

AS AN ADAPTOGEN, IT HELPS MANAGE STRESS, PROMOTES RESTFUL SLEEP, AND SUPPORTS ENERGY LEVELS DURING THE POSTPARTUM PERIOD, AIDING IN EMOTIONAL AND PHYSICAL RECOVERY.
IT IS COMMONLY TAKEN AS A TEA, IN CAPSULES, OR MIXED INTO FOOD FOR DAILY SUPPORT.

ASTRAGALUS
Astagalus membranaceus

STRENGTHENS THE IMMUNE SYSTEM, BOOSTS ENERGY, AND HELPS THE BODY RECOVER FROM THE STRESS OF CHILDBIRTH BY RESTORING QI (VITAL ENERGY). IT IS OFTEN CONSUMED AS A TEA, TINCTURE, OR ADDED TO SOUPS AND BROTHS FOR ITS RESTORATIVE PROPERTIES.

AVOCADO
Persea americana

THE LEAVES SUPPORT DIGESTIVE HEALTH, AID IN RESPIRATORY RECOVERY, AND PROVIDE A GENTLE DIURETIC EFFECT, HELPING TO REDUCE POSTPARTUM SWELLING. THEY ARE TYPICALLY BREWED AS A TEA OR INCLUDED IN HERBAL INFUSIONS.

CACAO
Theobrama cacao

CACAO CAN PROMOTE OXYTOCIN AND DOPAMINE SECRETION IN THE BRAIN WHICH CONTRIBUTES TO THE BONDING BETWEEN PARENT AND BABY. IT IS A SMOOTH-MUSCLE RELAXANT, AND MILD STIMULANT. IT PROVIDES AN OVERALL SENSE OF WELL-BEING, RELAXES THE WOMB, AND HELPS TO PREVENT PAINFUL AFTERBIRTH PAINS.
IT CAN BE TAKEN IN AN *ATOLE* (A TRADITIONAL MEXICAN DRINK MADE FROM CORNMEAL) OR WITH A POSTPARTUM INFUSION. TRADITIONALLY USED IN LABOR AND POSTPARTUM TO CALM, RELAX, AND NURTURE THE BIRTHING PERSON.

CINNAMON
Cinnamomum verum

CINNAMON IS WARMING, SUPPORTS DIGESTION, AND HELPS BALANCE BLOOD SUGAR LEVELS, WHICH CAN BE CRUCIAL FOR STABILIZING ENERGY AND MOOD IN THE POSTPARTUM PERIOD. IT IS ADDED TO TEAS, FOODS, OR TAKEN AS A SUPPLEMENT TO ENHANCE FLAVOR AND PROMOTE HEALTH.

COCONUT
Cocos nucifera

COCONUT IS HYDRATING AND RICH IN HEALTHY FATS, PROVIDING ESSENTIAL NUTRIENTS AND ENERGY, WHICH ARE VITAL FOR RECOVERY AND LACTATION. CONSUMED AS COCONUT WATER FOR HYDRATION, COCONUT OIL IN COOKING, OR COCONUT MILK FOR ADDED NUTRITION.

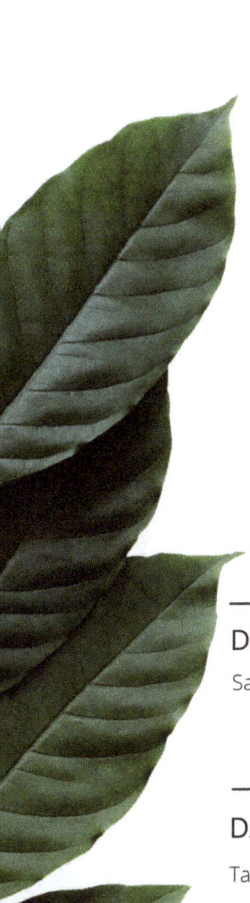

CRAMP BARK
Viburnum opulus

CRAMP BARK IS BENEFICIAL NOT ONLY FOR MENSTRUAL CRAMPS BUT ALSO FOR CRAMPS AND SPASMS ALL OVER THE BODY. IT MAY BE USED SPARINGLY FOR POSTPARTUM CRAMPING BUT IMPORTANT NOT TO INTERFERE TOO MUCH AS THESE CRAMPS ARE WORKING TO CLEANSE THE BODY AND SHRINK THE UTERUS BACK TO ITS NORMAL SIZE.

DAMIANA
Turnera diffusa

DAMIANA HAS A LONG TIME REPUTATION AS AN APHRODISIAC. THIS HERB BENEFITS WOMEN BY INCREASING BLOOD FLOW TO THE ABDOMEN AND GENITALS. IT ACTS AS A NATURAL MOOD ENHANCER AND RELAXANT, SUPPORTING EMOTIONAL BALANCE BY REDUCING ANXIETY AND MILD DEPRESSION THROUGH ITS CALMING AND UPLIFTING EFFECTS.

DAN SHEN
Salvia miltiorrhiza

DAN SHEN SUPPORTS BLOOD CIRCULATION, REDUCES INFLAMMATION, AND AIDS IN THE HEALING OF TISSUES AFTER CHILDBIRTH. IT IS OFTEN TAKEN AS A TEA, TINCTURE, OR IN DECOCTIONS AS PART OF A POSTPARTUM RECOVERY REGIMEN.

DANDELION
Taraxacum officinale

ROOT SUPPORTS LIVER HEALTH, AIDS DIGESTION, AND HELPS IN THE DETOXIFICATION PROCESS, WHICH CAN BE BENEFICIAL FOR A BODY RECOVERING FROM PREGNANCY AND BIRTH. COMMONLY TAKEN AS A TEA OR TINCTURE TO SUPPORT LIVER FUNCTION AND DIGESTION.

FENNEL
Foeniculum vulgare

FENNEL IS USED TO CALM STOMACH PAINS FROM CRAMPS AND CAESAREAN SECTION INDUCED GAS. IN NURSING, THIS HERB IS A COMMONLY KNOWN GALACTAGOGUE. ALTHOUGH THE ESSENTIAL OIL FOR THIS PLANT MAY BE TAKEN INTERNALLY AS A GALACTAGOGUE, THE SEED IS A MUCH SAFER OPTION FOR INGESTION.

FENUGREEK
Trigonella foenum-graeecum

FENUGREEK IS WELL-KNOWN FOR ITS ABILITY TO BOOST MILK PRODUCTION IN BREASTFEEDING MOTHERS AND ALSO SUPPORTS DIGESTION AND ENERGY LEVELS. IT IS TYPICALLY CONSUMED AS A TEA, IN FOOD, OR AS A SUPPLEMENT.

GINGER
Zingiber officinale

GINGER IS RENOWNED FOR ITS ABILITY TO SUPPORT DIGESTION, REDUCE INFLAMMATION, AND PROMOTE CIRCULATION, MAKING IT BENEFICIAL DURING THE POSTPARTUM PERIOD. IT IS COMMONLY CONSUMED AS A TEA, IN FOOD, OR AS A SUPPLEMENT.

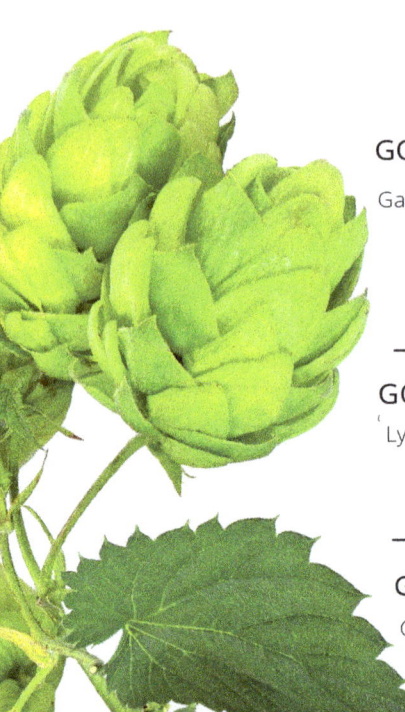

GOATS RUE
Galega officinalis

GOATS RUE IS AN ESSENTIAL GALACTAGOGUE USED TO PROMOTE MILK SUPPLY AND GROW GLANDULAR TISSUE IN THE BREASTS. THIS HERB IS APPLICABLE IN THE CASE OF TUBULAR HYPOPLASTIC BREASTS, FOR WOMEN LOOKING TO NURSE AN ADOPTED CHILD OR TO INCREASE GENERAL MILK SUPPLY. IT IS ALSO USED TO LOWER BLOOD SUGAR LEVELS IN NATURAL DIABETIC THERAPIES.

GOJI BERRY
Lycium barbarum

RICH IN ANTIOXIDANTS, SUPPORTS IMMUNE HEALTH, AND BOOSTS ENERGY, MAKING IT AN EXCELLENT ADDITION TO A POSTPARTUM RECOVERY REGIMEN. CONSUMED AS A SNACK, ADDED TO TEAS, OR USED IN SOUPS FOR ITS NOURISHING BENEFITS.

GOTU KOLA
Centella asiatica

GOTU KOLA IS A GREAT HERB FOR COGNITIVE FUNCTIONING AND OFTEN PAIRED WITH GINKGO. THE TOPICAL FORM OF THIS HERB HAS ALSO BEEN FOUND TO DECREASE C-SECTION WOUND HEALING TIME.

GUAVA
Psidium guajava

GUAVA LEAVES HELP REDUCE INFLAMMATION, AID IN UTERINE HEALTH, AND SUPPORT DIGESTION, MAKING THEM VALUABLE FOR POSTPARTUM RECOVERY.
TYPICALLY BREWED AS A TEA OR USED IN BATHS AND STEAMS TO HARNESS THEIR HEALING PROPERTIES.

HOLY BASIL
Ocimum sanctum

HOLY BASIL IS A CRUCIAL ADAPTOGEN IN AYURVEDA. IT HELPS THE BODY RESTORE BALANCE AFTER A STRESSFUL SITUATION MAKING IT GREAT FOR USE AFTER BIRTH. THIS HERB MAY BE TAKEN ROUTINELY OVER A LONG PERIOD OF TIME AS A TONIC.

HOPS
Humulus lupulus

HOPS IS A GREAT HERB TO TRY FOR THOSES HAVING TROUBLE SLEEPING. IT MAY ALSO BE USED AS A NERVOUS SYSTEM TONIC. MOST PEOPLE USE THIS HERB AS A TINCTURE, HOWEVER, TEA FORM WORKS WELL TOO IF YOU DON'T MIND THE TASTE. HOPS ARE ALSO AN ESSENTIAL AND LONG-STORIED GALACTAGOGUE.

JUJUBEE
Ziziphus jujuba

JUJUBE NOURISHES THE BLOOD, BOOSTS ENERGY, AND SUPPORTS DIGESTION, ALL OF WHICH ARE CRUCIAL DURING THE POSTPARTUM PERIOD TO RESTORE VITALITY AND BALANCE. CONSUMED AS A SNACK, ADDED TO SOUPS, OR BREWED AS A TEA FOR ITS SWEET, NOURISHING BENEFITS.

KATRAFRAY
Catgenus spegazzinii

BARK REDUCES INFLAMMATION, RELIEVES PAIN, AND SUPPORTS SKIN HEALING, OFFERING RELIEF FROM COMMON POSTPARTUM ACHES AND PAINS.
OFTEN USED AS AN ESSENTIAL OIL OR IN HERBAL BATHS TO SOOTHE THE BODY AND PROMOTE RECOVERY.

LAVENDER
Lavandula angustifolia

LAVENDER IS SHOWN TO BE HELPFUL FOR TENSION HEADACHE, IT ALSO PROMOTES CALM FEELINGS NEEDED FOR A GOOD NIGHTS SLEEP. THIS HERB HAS BEEN USED FOR DEPRESSION AND DURING THE POSTPARTUM TIME OF HORMONAL SHIFTS. ADDITIONALLY, WHEN LAVENDER IS HARVESTED AT ITS PEAK MEDICINAL POTENCY, IT HAS BEEN KNOWN TO SOOTHE DIGESTION.

MARSHMALLOW
Althaea officinalis

MARSHMALLOW IS ONE OF THE BEST MUCILAGINOUS HERBS. THE HERB IS GREAT ON AREAS OF INFLAMMATION INTERNALLY AS WELL AS EXTERNALLY. MARSHMALLOW ADDITIONALLY WORKS WELL IN AIDING THE LUNGS AND URINARY TRACT.

MORINGA
Moringa oleifera

PREVIOUS STUDIES HAVE SHOWN THAT GIVING MORINGA LEAF TO PREGNANT WOMEN INCREASES THE LEVEL OF IRON IN THEIR BODY. STUDIES ALSO SHOW THAT INTAKE OF MORINGA LEAF PREVENTS ANEMIA, IMPROVES THE QUANTITY OF MILK AND THE WELL-BEING OF THE BREASTFEEDING MOTHER. ONLY USE THE LEAVES. AVOID THE FLOWER AND SEED DURING PREGNANCY AND POSTPARTUM.

NETTLE
Urtica dioica

RICH IN IRON AND OTHER ESSENTIAL NUTRIENTS, MAKING IT EXCELLENT FOR REBUILDING BLOOD AND ENERGY LEVELS, AS WELL AS SUPPORTING OVERALL RECOVERY. TYPICALLY BREWED AS A TEA OR ADDED TO SOUPS AND STEWS TO SUPPORT POSTPARTUM HEALING.

OATS
Avena sativa

OATS PROVIDE NOURISHING SUPPORT FOR ENERGY LEVELS AND SOOTHE THE NERVOUS SYSTEM, MAKING THEM IDEAL FOR PROMOTING RELAXATION AND RECOVERY. HOW TO USE: CONSUMED AS OATMEAL, OAT MILK, OR IN HERBAL TEAS FOR A CALMING, NUTRITIOUS BOOST.

PAPAYA
Carica papaya

PAPAYA, RICH IN VITAMINS A, C, AND E, FOLATE, FIBER, AND DIGESTIVE ENZYMES LIKE PAPAIN, SUPPORTS DIGESTION, PREVENTS CONSTIPATION, AND BOOSTS IMMUNITY DURING POSTPARTUM RECOVERY. ITS ANTI-INFLAMMATORY PROPERTIES HELP REDUCE SWELLING AND PROMOTE HEALING. PAPAYA CAN BE EATEN FRESH, BLENDED INTO SMOOTHIES, ADDED TO SALADS, OR BREWED AS TEA FROM ITS LEAVES. THE RIPE PULP CAN ALSO BE USED AS A POULTICE TO SOOTHE INFLAMMATION AND AID WOUND HEALING.

PARTRIDGE BERRY
Mitchella repens

PARTRIDGE BERRY IS VERY GOOD FOR TONING AND NOURISHING THE UTERUS. IT IS OFTEN INCLUDED IN FORMULAS TO PREVENT MISCARRIAGES. THIS HERB IS USEFUL FOR INFERTILITY DUE TO HORMONE IMBALANCES, STOPS HEMORRHAGE, AS WELL AS SUPPORTS AND NOURISHES THE UTERUS ENABLING A SUCCESSFUL LABOR.

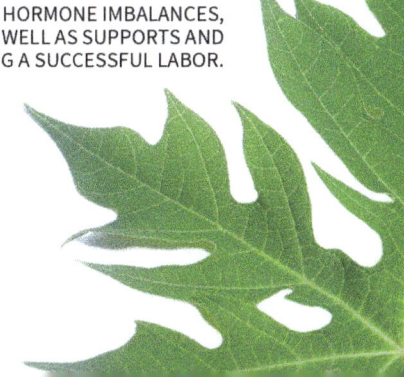

PLANTAIN

Plantago major

KNOWN FOR ITS WOUND-HEALING PROPERTIES, SOOTHING INFLAMMATION, AND SUPPORTING DIGESTIVE HEALTH, ALL OF WHICH ARE BENEFICIAL DURING POSTPARTUM RECOVERY. APPLIED TOPICALLY AS A POULTICE OR TAKEN AS A TEA OR INFUSION TO AID IN HEALING.

RED RASPBERRY

Rubus idaeus

TONES THE UTERUS, SUPPORTS UTERINE RECOVERY, AND AIDS IN BALANCING HORMONES, MAKING IT A STAPLE IN POSTPARTUM CARE. IT IS COMMONLY BREWED AS A TEA OR TAKEN IN CAPSULE FORM FOR ITS TONING AND NOURISHING EFFECTS.

ROSE

Rosa spp.

ROSE IS HIGH IN PREBIOTICS, SOOTHING, AND AN ASTRINGENT. IT IS CALMING, GREAT FOR HEMORRHOIDS, EMOTIONALLY DRAINING OR TRAUMATIC BIRTHS, AND DIGESTIVE IMBALANCES. IF YOU ARE FEELING CONSTIPATED OR BLOATED AFTER BIRTH, OR IF BABY IS COLICKY, TAKE THIS INFUSION THREE TIMES A DAY. ROSE IS ALSO USED IN WASHES/RINSES, BATHS, AND VAGINAL STEAMS.

SCHIZANDRA

Schisandra chinensis

AN ADAPTOGEN THAT SUPPORTS STRESS REDUCTION, LIVER FUNCTION, AND OVERALL VITALITY, HELPING NEW MOTHERS COPE WITH THE PHYSICAL AND EMOTIONAL DEMANDS OF POSTPARTUM LIFE. BERRIES TYPICALLY TAKEN AS A TEA, TINCTURE, OR IN POWDERED FORM TO SUPPORT RECOVERY.

SEA MOSS

Chondrus crispus

SEA MOSS CAN PROVIDE THE BODY WITH A LOT OF VITAMINS AND MINERALS. THESE NUTRIENTS INCLUDE IODINE, CALCIUM, B VITAMINS, AND ZINC. IT IS ALSO FULL OF PREBIOTIC AND HAS ANTI-INFLAMMATORY, ANTIMICROBIAL PROPERTIES. ITS MUCILAGE CONTENT AIDS IN EASING BOWEL MOVEMENTS.

SLIPPERY ELM

Ulmus rubra

SLIPPERY ELM IS A HIGHLY NUTRITIOUS HERB DUE TO ITS HIGH MUCILAGE CONTENT. THIS HERB WORKS VERY WELL FOR INFLAMED AND IRRITATED MUCUS MEMBRANES. WHEN TAKEN ORALLY, IT HAS BEEN SEEN TO HELP WITH DIGESTIVE ISSUES, COUGHS, AS WELL AS SORE THROATS.

TURMERIC

Curcuma longa

A POWERFUL ANTI-INFLAMMATORY THAT SUPPORTS HEALING, IMMUNE FUNCTION, AND OVERALL RECOVERY, MAKING IT BENEFICIAL FOR POSTPARTUM CARE. CONSUMED IN FOOD, AS GOLDEN MILK, OR AS A TEA TO ENHANCE ITS HEALING EFFECTS.

YELLOW DOCK

Rumex crispus

YELLOW DOCK IS HELPFUL FOR ANEMIA OR CONSTIPATION. THE HERB IS HIGH IN IRON AND TANNINS. THIS HERB CLEANSES THE BLOOD AND IMPROVES LIVER HEALTH. THIS IS A GREAT IRON SUPPLEMENT OR LAXATIVE DURING PREGNANCY OR NURSING DUE TO ITS GENTLE AND NUTRITIONAL COMPONENTS.

"The unsupported new mother is the most tragic thing on the planet."

-Yosara
Birth Advocate

AFTERBIRTH CHILLS & SWEATING

AFTER-PAINS ARE CONTRACTIONS THAT OCCUR AFTER LABOR AND DELIVERY. THESE CONTRACTIONS SIGNAL THE PROCESS OF INVOLUTION, THE PROCESS OF THE UTERUS SHRINKING BACK DOWN TO ITS PRE-PREGNANCY SIZE AND SHAPE. AFTERPAINS BEGIN AROUND 12 HOURS AFTER BIRTH. RANGING FROM MILD DISCOMFORT TO INTENSE PAIN FOR SOME. THEY USUALLY BECOME MORE INTENSE DURING FUTURE BIRTHS BECAUSE THE UTERUS GENERALLY BECOMES MORE STRETCHED WITH EACH PREGNANCY. THEY OFTEN CEASE WITHIN 72 HOURS AFTER BIRTH. THESE PAINS ARE PURPOSEFUL. SO IT IS IMPORTANT TO USE COMFORT MEASURES SPARINGLY IN THIS CASE.

HERBS/REMEDIES: ALLEVIATES AFTER-PAINS, SUPPORTS UTERINE RECOVERY, SOOTHES DISCOMFORT, AND ENHANCES OVERALL POSTPARTUM COMFORT.

TINCTURE:
1 PART CRAMP BARK
½ PART GINGER
¼ PART BLACK COHOSH
¼ PART MOTHERWORT
1 TSP UP TO 4X DAILY EITHER IN PLAIN WATER OR ADDED TO TEA

TEA
1 PART CRAMP BARK
½ PART GINGER
¼ PART GINSENG

DRINK 1-4 CUPS A DAY

TEA
1 PART CATNIP
1 PART NETTLE
½ PART CHAMOMILE
1/8 PART LAVENDER
DRINK 1-4 CUPS A DAY

HEAT PACKS
MOXIEBUSTION AND RICE PACKS

MOTHER ROASTING, A PRACTICE ROOTED IN THE MANY TRADITIONS INCLUDING THOSE OF SOUTHERN BLACK MIDWIVES, IS A POSTPARTUM CARE TECHNIQUE THAT EMPHASIZES WARMING AND COMFORTING THE NEW MOTHER. THIS PRACTICE INVOLVES USING HEAT TO HELP THE MOTHER RECOVER FROM CHILDBIRTH, BOTH PHYSICALLY AND EMOTIONALLY. TRADITIONALLY, IT INCLUDES PLACING WARM COMPRESSES OR HEATED STONES WRAPPED IN CLOTHS AROUND THE MOTHER'S ABDOMEN, LOWER BACK, AND OTHER AREAS THAT MAY BE SORE OR TENSE. THE HEAT IS BELIEVED TO PROMOTE RELAXATION, EASE MUSCLE TENSION, AND SUPPORT UTERINE CONTRACTION AND HEALING. IN ADDITION TO THE PHYSICAL BENEFITS, MOTHER ROASTING IS A RITUAL THAT FOSTERS EMOTIONAL SUPPORT AND BONDING, REFLECTING THE COMMUNITY-CENTERED APPROACH OF SOUTHERN BLACK MIDWIFERY PRACTICES. THIS NURTURING TECHNIQUE HONORS THE MOTHER'S TRANSITION INTO POSTPARTUM AND HELPS TO ENSURE A SMOOTH AND SUPPORTIVE RECOVERY PERIOD.

BACKACHE POST EPIDURAL

THIS TINCTURE ALLEVIATES BACK PAIN FOLLOWING AN EPIDURAL, REDUCES INFLAMMATION, SUPPORTS MUSCLE RELAXATION, AND AIDS IN RECOVERY. USE IN MODERATION, ESPECIALLY WHEN BREASTFEEDING.

HERBS/REMEDIES: SUPPORTS POST-EPIDURAL BACK PAIN, EASES MUSCLE TENSION, SUPPORTS SPINAL RECOVERY, AND HELPS MANAGE DISCOMFORT.

TINCTURE:
- ½ OZ CRAMP BARK
- ¼ OZ BLACK COHOSH
- ¼ OZ MOTHERWORT

USE UP TO 4 TIMES DAILY, EITHER IN PLAIN WATER OR ADDED TO TEA

HERBS/REMEDIES: REDUCE PAIN AND MUSCLE TENSION, AND SUPPORTS SPINAL RECOVERY

TEA
- 1 PART CALIFORNIA POPPY
- ¼ PART NETTLE
- 1 TBL PER CUP OF WATER. STEEP FOR 30 MINUTES UP TO OVERNIGHT DRINK UP TO 1 QUART DAILY

CESAREAN INCISION

THIS HERBAL OIL* IS DESIGNED TO SUPPORT POSTPARTUM RECOVERY BY REPLENISHING ESSENTIAL NUTRIENTS, TONING THE UTERUS, BOOSTING IMMUNITY, AND SOOTHING DIGESTION.

HERBS/REMEDIES: SUPPORTS HEALING OF C-SECTION INCISIONS, REDUCES INFLAMMATION, AND PROMOTES SKIN REGENERATION. APPLY THE OIL BLEND TO THE INCISION AREA REGULARLY FOR OPTIMAL RECOVERY.

INFUSE
- 1 PART GOTA KOLA
- ¼ PART MUGWORT
- ¼ PART ST JOHNS WORT
- CASTOR OIL (VOLUME IS BASED ON YOUR DESIRED AMOUNT)

COMBINE YOUR CHOSEN HERBS WITH THE OIL IN A CLEAN, DRY JAR, ENSURING THE HERBS ARE FULLY SUBMERGED, THEN SEAL THE JAR AND LET IT SIT IN A WARM, SUNNY SPOT FOR 1 TO 2 WEEKS, SHAKING GENTLY DAILY; STRAIN THE MIXTURE THROUGH A FINE MESH STRAINER OR CHEESECLOTH BEFORE USE.

OR USING A DOUBLE BOILER, PLACE A HEATPROOF BOWL OR SMALLER POT WITH THE OIL AND HERBS OVER A LARGER POT OF SIMMERING WATER, ENSURING THE BOTTOM OF THE BOWL DOES NOT TOUCH THE WATER, AND GENTLY HEAT THE MIXTURE FOR 1 TO 2 HOURS, STIRRING OCCASIONALLY TO ALLOW THE HERBAL PROPERTIES TO FULLY INFUSE INTO THE OIL.

*OIL CAN ALSO BE MADE INTO A SALVE BY ADDING BEESWAX.

BEGIN USING ONCE WOUND HAS FULLY CLOSED AND THE STITCHES OR STAPLES HAVE BEEN REMOVED (TYPICALLY AROUND 1 TO 2 WEEKS AFTER SURGERY). ENSURE THE INCISION IS CLEAN, DRY, AND FREE FROM ANY SIGNS OF INFECTION BEFORE APPLYING TOPICAL TREATMENTS. APPLY THE OIL BLEND TO THE INCISION AREA FOR OPTIMAL RECOVERY.

POSTPARTUM SITZ BATH

SOOTHING BLEND THAT AIDS IN HEALING AFTER CHILDBIRTH
HERBS/REMEDIES: ANTI-INFLAMMATORY, ANTI-MICROBIAL, AND VULNERARY SUPPORT

POSTPARTUM SITZ BATH:
- 1 PART CALENDULA
- 1 PART WITCH HAZEL
- 1 PART COMFREY LEAVES
- ½ PART ROSE
- ¼ PART EPSOLM SALT

ADD HOT WATER AND STEEP FOR 20 MINUTES. STRAIN, AND PLACE IN SITZ BASIN

POSTPARTUM BLEEDING

POSTPARTUM BLEEDING AND UTERINE RECOVERY ARE COMMON CONCERNS AFTER CHILDBIRTH, WITH THE BODY NEEDING SUPPORT AT TIMES TO MANAGE BLEEDING AND SUPPORT UTERINE HEALTH. IN EMERGENCY SITUATIONS A TRAINED PRACTITIONER SHOULD BE CONSULTED.

HERBS/REMEDIES: SHEPHERD'S PURSE FOR REDUCING BLEEDING, RASPBERRY LEAF FOR UTERINE HEALTH, AND OPTIONAL SPEARMINT FOR FLAVOR AND DIGESTION.

STYPIC TEA:
- ½ PART SHEPHERDS PURSE
- ½ PART RASPBERRY LEAF
- ¼ PART SPEARMINT

STEEP 4 TEASPOONS OF THE BLEND IN HOT WATER FOR 20 MINUTES. STRAIN, MAY HAVE UP TO 4 CUPS DAILY.

POSTPARTUM MOOD

AIDS IN CALMING THE NERVOUS SYSTEM, REDUCING STRESS, AND PROMOTING OVERALL EMOTIONAL WELL-BEING.

HERBS/REMEDIES: THIS BLEND SUPPORTS MOOD STABILIZATION AND HORMONE BALANCE DURING POSTPARTUM RECOVERY.

TINCTURE:
- 2 PART MOTHERWORT TINCTURE
- 1 PART VITEX TINCTURE
- ½ PART BLUE VERVAIN TINCTURE
- ½ PART HOLY BASIL TINCTURE
- ½ PART SKULLCAP TINCTURE
- ½ PART ASHWAGANDA TINCTURE

TAKE ½ TO 1 TSP AS NEEDED UP TO 4 TSP DAILY FOR 2 WEEKS

COMFORT & CALM TEA
- 1 PART LEMON BALM
- 1 PART HOLY BASIL
- ½ PART MOTHERWORT
- ½ PART BLUE VERVAIN
- ¼ SPRINKLE OF ROSES

INFUSE 1 TBL TO 8 OZ OF WATER. DRINK 1-4 CUPS A DAY.

POSTPARTUM PAIN AND SLEEP

THIS TINCTURE SOOTHES ANXIETY, PROMOTES RESTFUL SLEEP, RELIEVES MUSCLE TENSION AND UTERINE CRAMPS. USE IN MODERATION, ESPECIALLY WHEN BREASTFEEDING

HERBS/REMEDIES: REDUCES STRESS, ENHANCES RELAXATION, IMPROVES SLEEP QUALITY, REDUCES RESTLESSNESS, CALMS NERVES, HORMONAL SHIFTS, PHYSICAL RECOVERY

TINCTURE:
- 1 PART CALIFORNIA POPPY
- 1 PART CRAMP BARK
- 1 PART PASSION FLOWER
- ½ PART HOPS
- ¼ PART CHAMOMILE
- ¼ PART GLYCERIN

FOLLOW TINCTURE MAKING DIRECTIONS IN HERBAL PREPARATIONS CHAPTER. TAKE 1-2 DROPPERS FULL IN A SMALL AMOUNT OF WATER OR JUICE BEFORE BED TO HELP WITH PAIN AND SLEEP.

POSTPARTUM SUPPORT TEA

THIS HERBAL TEA BLEND IS DESIGNED TO SUPPORT POSTPARTUM RECOVERY BY REPLENISHING ESSENTIAL NUTRIENTS, TONING THE UTERUS, BOOSTING IMMUNITY, AND SOOTHING DIGESTION.

HERBS/REMEDIES: NETTLE LEAF IS RICH IN IRON AND CALCIUM, ALFALFA PROVIDES ESSENTIAL VITAMINS AND MINERALS FOR STRENGTH, ROSE HIPS BOOST IMMUNITY WITH VITAMIN C, SPEARMINT AIDS DIGESTION, AND RED RASPBERRY LEAF TONES THE UTERUS TO SUPPORT POSTPARTUM HEALING.

- 1 PART NETTLE LEAF
- ½ PART ALFALFA
- ½ PART LEMON BALM
- ½ PART ROSE HIPS
- ½ PART SPEARMINT
- ¼ PART ROSE BUDS

1 TBL PER CUP OF WATER. STEEP FOR 30 MINUTES UP TO OVERNIGHT. DRINK UP TO 1 QUART DAILY

"In every drop of breast milk, a mother offers her child the protection of her ancestors."

— Valerie Goodness, Lakota Midwife

chapter 7

Breastfeeding
Galactagogues
Weaning
Lactation Support Recipes
Usage Guide For Nursing Through

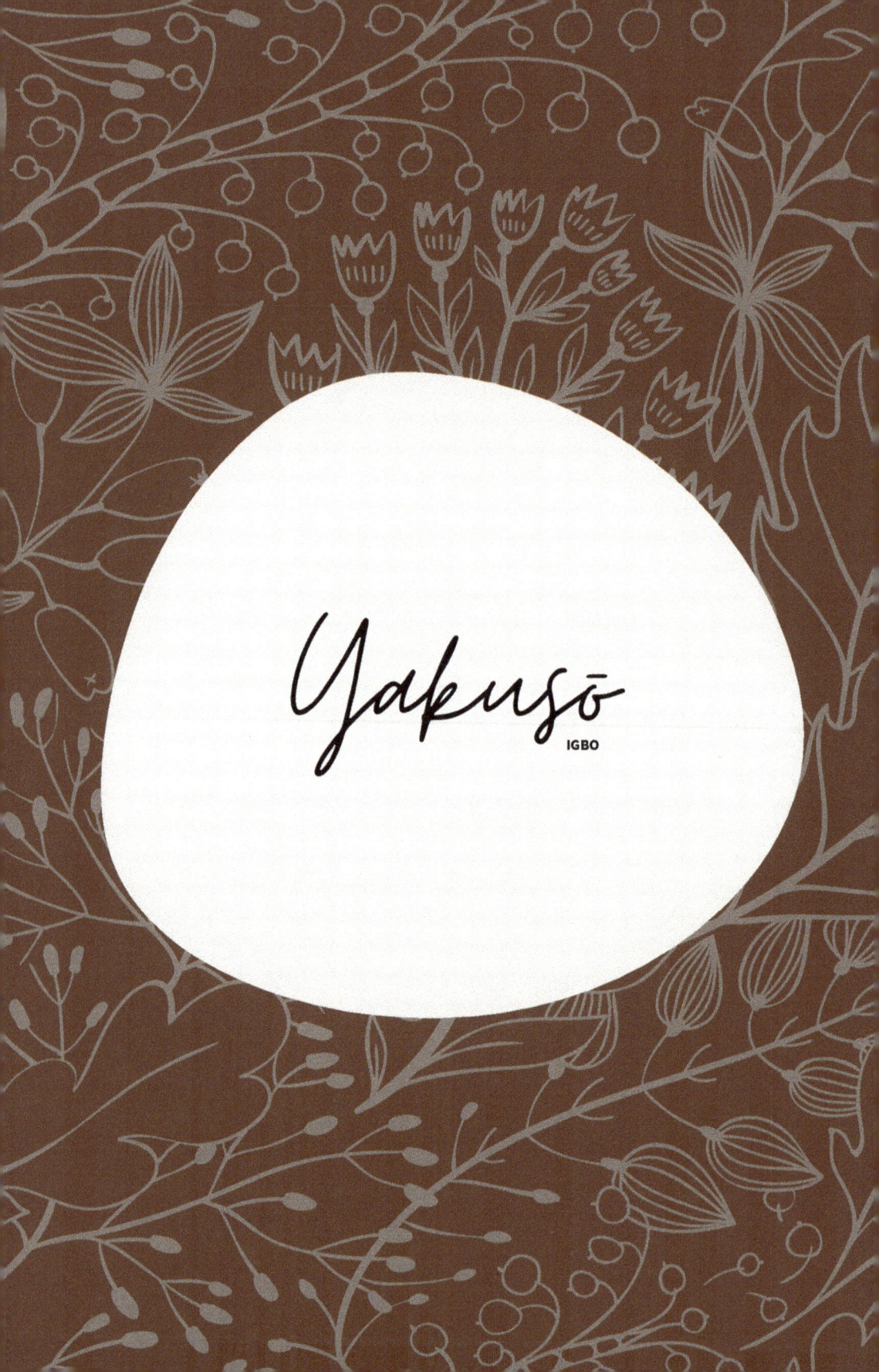

The Sacred Bond: Perspectives on Breastfeeding and Holistic Postpartum Care

In Indigenous cultures, breastfeeding is revered as a deeply spiritual and essential part of holistic postpartum care. It is seen as an extension of the sacred bond formed in the womb, where the mother's body continues to nourish and protect her child in the physical world. Breastfeeding is more than a means of providing sustenance; it is the transference of ancestral wisdom, love, and strength to the baby. Through this act, a mother imparts the teachings of her lineage, ensuring that her child is connected to the traditions, values, and spirits of her people.

Breastfeeding is also understood as a vital component of the baby's overall well-being. It is believed to fortify the child not just physically, but also emotionally and spiritually. The act of breastfeeding helps to ground the baby in the world, providing comfort and security as they adjust to life outside the womb. This nurturing process is seen as an investment in the future, ensuring that the child grows strong, healthy, and rooted in the cultural and spiritual teachings of their community.

In many Indigenous communities, breastfeeding is not the sole responsibility of the mother but is supported by a network of women—grandmothers, aunties, sisters, and other community members—who offer guidance, assistance, and encouragement. This collective support reflects the belief that the well-being of the child is intertwined with the well-being of the community. If a mother is unable to breastfeed, it is not seen as a failure. Instead, other mothers in the community may step in to nurse the baby, demonstrating the communal nature of child-rearing and the shared responsibility for the child's health and growth.

It is also recognized that not every mother can or chooses to breastfeed, and within Indigenous cultures, this choice is respected. Motherhood is honored in its many forms, and the love and care a mother provides are what truly define her role. The community ensures that every mother and child is supported, regardless of their breastfeeding experience.

Indigenous postpartum care is holistic, encompassing the physical, emotional, and spiritual needs of both mother and child. Breastfeeding is one of the many ways in which this care is provided, carrying forward the wisdom and strength of generations while nurturing the next. The deep reverence for this practice is a testament to the understanding that in nurturing the mother and child, the future of the community is also nurtured.

Realities of Breastfeeding

Breastfeeding is often portrayed as a natural, effortless process, yet many women face significant challenges in their breastfeeding journeys. Modern culture can impose dangerously high expectations, making it seem like breastfeeding should be easy and instinctive. This misconception can leave new parents feeling inadequate, as though they should automatically know how to breastfeed without support or guidance.

Breastfeeding is a learning process for both the mother and the baby. After an intense birth experience, both need to figure out how to work together to establish a successful breastfeeding routine. It's important to recognize that breastfeeding, like learning to walk, requires time and patience while the mother and baby adapt to each other's needs and signals.

The myth that breastfeeding should come naturally can lead to feelings of insufficiency. Many parents struggle to find their rhythm and may need assistance to navigate this complex process. Seeking help from an IBCLC, International Board-Certified Lactation Consultant, or local breastfeeding support groups can provide guidance and encouragement.

It is crucial to avoid comparisons and shaming, as these can add unnecessary pressure. The most important aspect of breastfeeding is establishing a proper latch, which is essential for preventing nipple injury and ensuring a good milk supply. The latch takes priority over the use of galactagogues (milk-boosting herbs or foods) because a correct latch will support effective milk transfer and minimize discomfort.

The process of breastfeeding is filled with unique aspects that make it a magical experience. For instance, the areola darkens during pregnancy to help guide the baby's limited vision, and it may even have a scent reminiscent of amniotic fluid, which helps the baby feel connected to their recent home. Additionally, signals from the baby's immune system can influence the composition of breast milk, providing tailored support for the baby's health. Breast milk also varies throughout the day; it may be richer in certain nutrients in the morning and have different properties at night.

Breastfeeding offers many benefits for mothers, including supporting postpartum recovery through uterine contractions and lowering the risk of certain cancers, while strengthening the bond between mother and baby. Remember, the length of time you breastfeed should make sense for both you and your baby, there's no one-size-fits-all approach. Above all, be gentle with yourself. Breastfeeding is a journey that takes time, patience, and practice. With the right support, you'll discover what works best for you and your baby

"In our village, a child fed at the breast is considered blessed by the gods."

— Latin American Saying

Galactagogues

A galactagogue is a substance, often an herb or food, that is believed to increase milk supply in breastfeeding mothers. These substances can stimulate or enhance the production of breast milk, supporting lactation during times when milk supply might be low or when the mother desires to increase her supply.

Examples of Galactagogues:

Fenugreek *(Trigonella foenum-graecum)*
Usage: Take 1-2 capsules (580-610 mg) 3 times daily or decoct 1 teaspoon of fenugreek seeds in hot water to make tea.
Contraindications: Not recommended for women with diabetes, as it can lower blood sugar levels. Avoid if allergic to peanuts or chickpeas.
Notes: May cause a maple syrup-like odor in urine and sweat. Fenugreek may cause gas in some people and breastfeeding babies. If this occurs, discontinue use.

Oatmeal *(Avena sativa)*
Usage: Consume as part of your daily diet, in the form of oatmeal, oat cookies, or oat milk.
Contraindications: Generally safe, but large amounts may cause bloating or gas in sensitive individuals.
Notes: Also a great source of iron, which can support energy levels postpartum.

Fennel *(Foeniculum vulgare)*
Usage: Brew 1-2 teaspoons of fennel seeds in hot water to make tea, or use fennel oil (diluted) in cooking.
Contraindications: Avoid if you have a history of seizures or allergic reactions to celery or carrots.
Notes: Also helps with digestion and reducing colic in babies.

Shatavari *(Asparagus racemosus)*
Usage: Take 1-2 teaspoons of powdered root daily, mixed with milk or water.
Contraindications: Avoid if you have a known allergy to asparagus. Consult with a healthcare provider if you have a hormonal imbalance.
Notes: Also supports reproductive health and hormonal balance.

Alfalfa (Medicago sativa)
Usage: Take 1-2 capsules (500 mg) 3 times daily or use fresh alfalfa sprouts in salads.
Contraindications: Avoid if you have lupus or other autoimmune conditions.
Notes: Also a good source of vitamins and minerals.

Goat's Rue *(Galega officinalis)*
Usage: Take 1-2 capsules (300-500 mg) 3 times daily or brew 1 teaspoon of dried leaves in hot water for tea.
Contraindications: Not recommended during pregnancy. Consult a healthcare provider if you have diabetes.
Notes: Works by stimulating the growth of mammary glands. It contains compounds believed to have galactagogue properties, which promote milk production and can support the development of breast tissue, making it particularly useful for breastfeeding mothers who want to increase milk supply.

Blessed Thistle *(Cnicus benedictus)*
Usage: Take 1-2 capsules (390 mg) 3 times daily or steep 1 teaspoon in a cup of boiling water for tea.
Contraindications: Should not be used during pregnancy. Consult a healthcare provider if you have a history of stomach ulcers.
Notes: Often combined with fenugreek.

Brewer's Yeast *(Saccharomyces cerevisiae)*
Usage: Add 1-2 tablespoons to food or smoothies daily.
Contraindications: May cause bloating or gas. Avoid if you have a yeast allergy.
Notes: Rich in B vitamins, which can support overall energy and mood.

Anise *(Pimpinella anisum)*
Usage: Brew 1-2 teaspoons of anise seeds in hot water to make tea.
Contraindications: Avoid in large amounts as it can be toxic. Not recommended for use in pregnancy.
Notes: Helps with digestion and can reduce colic in babies.

Milk Thistle *(Silybum marianum)*
Usage: Take 1-2 capsules (200-400 mg) 3 times daily or brew seeds in hot water for tea.
Contraindications: Consult a healthcare provider if you have a history of hormone-sensitive conditions.
Notes: Also supports liver health.

The Latch

Ensuring a correct latch is one of the most crucial factors in successful breastfeeding. While galactagogues—herbs and foods that promote milk production can be supportive, they are not a substitute for a proper latch. A correct latch allows the baby to effectively extract milk, stimulates milk production, and helps prevent common issues such as sore nipples, blocked ducts, or insufficient milk supply. Without this foundation, even the most potent galactagogues may not be effective, as milk production is primarily driven by the demand created by the baby's suckling.

When considering the use of galactagogues, it is essential to prioritize establishing and maintaining a correct latch. Galactagogues can be beneficial, but they should complement—not replace—the foundational aspects of breastfeeding. If the process is challenging, it is highly encouraged to seek help from a lactation consultant to ensure the best outcomes for both mother and baby.

Beyond its role as nourishment, breast milk is often referred to as "liquid gold" for its incredible nutritional and healing properties, extending far beyond just feeding. Many parents creatively use breast milk to support their baby's health in various ways. For instance, adding a small amount of breast milk to a baby's bath can help soothe and moisturize sensitive skin, providing relief from rashes or dryness. Additionally, breast milk can be used to create nourishing baby body butter by mixing it with natural oils like coconut or shea butter, offering protection and hydration for delicate skin.

Breast milk body butter is a unique product made by combining breast milk with oils and butters like coconut oil, shea butter, or cocoa butter to create a moisturizing blend. To stabilize the mixture, an emulsifier such as beeswax is often used to blend the water content in breast milk with the oils. These practices leverage the milk's natural antibodies, enzymes, and fatty acids, making breast milk a gentle and effective remedy for various skin concerns. However, breast milk is highly perishable due to its water content and nutrient-rich composition, making it prone to bacterial growth. Even with preservatives, its shelf life is limited, and careful handling is essential to ensure safety and hygiene. By using breast milk in these creative ways, parents can maximize its benefits.

Weaning

Weaning is a personal journey, and there is no right or wrong way to go about it. Whether you are returning to work, no longer enjoying the process, or your baby has decided they are no longer interested, trust your instincts, be gentle with yourself, and allow the process to unfold at a pace that feels right for both you and your child.

Suggestions for Weaning:

1. Gradual Reduction: Start by dropping one nursing session at a time, giving your body and your baby time to adjust. Typically, you can start with the least favorite feeding of the day, often mid-day.
2. Offer Alternatives: As you reduce breastfeeding sessions, offer your baby other forms of nourishment like formula, cow's milk (if they are over one year old), or solid foods. This can be paired with comfort items like a favorite blanket or a cuddly toy to provide emotional support.
3. Comfort Measures: If your breasts become engorged, consider expressing just enough milk to relieve discomfort. Homeopathic and herbal remedies, such as pain and inflammation relief blends, lymphatic support, and compresses, along with over-the-counter pain relievers, may also be helpful.
4. Distraction: Engage your baby in fun activities or outings during the times they would typically nurse. This can help them focus on other things and gradually forget about breastfeeding.
5. Night Weaning: Nighttime feedings can be the hardest to let go of, both for you and your baby. If your baby is waking up to nurse out of habit rather than hunger, you can gradually offer an alternative, like a soothing back rub, instead of nursing. It may take time and patience, but eventually, your baby will adjust to the new routine.

Weaning can bring a mix of emotions, from relief to sadness. It is normal to grieve the end of this special chapter, even if you are ready to move on. Creating a ritual or ceremony to commemorate the time spent breastfeeding can be healing. Consider writing a letter to your child, creating a memory box with items related to your breastfeeding journey, or even crafting a small trophy to celebrate the accomplishment.

Remember, the bond you have established through breastfeeding will sustain long after the feedings have ended. This bond is not defined solely by nursing, or how long you nursed, but by the love, care, and connection you share with your child every day.

LACTATION SUPPORT TEA

THIS HERBAL TEA BLEND IS CRAFTED TO ENHANCE MILK PRODUCTION, NOURISH THE BODY, AND PROMOTE CALMNESS DURING BREASTFEEDING.

HERBS/REMEDIES:
MORINGA IS A NUTRIENT POWERHOUSE THAT BOOSTS OVERALL HEALTH AND MILK SUPPLY, WHILE GOAT'S RUE TRADITIONALLY STIMULATES LACTATION AND SUPPORTS MAMMARY TISSUE. ALFALFA PROVIDES ESSENTIAL VITAMINS AND MINERALS FOR LACTATION, SPEARMINT AIDS DIGESTION WITH A REFRESHING FLAVOR, AND OAT TOPS ARE RICH IN MINERALS THAT SUPPORT THE NERVOUS SYSTEM AND ENCOURAGE MILK FLOW.

TEA
- 1 PART MORINGA
- ½ PART GOAT'S RUE
- ½ PART ALFALFA
- 1 PART SPEARMINT
- ¼ PART OAT TOPS

INSTRUCTIONS:
USE 1 TABLESPOON OF THE BLEND PER CUP OF WATER. STEEP FOR 30 MINUTES OR UP TO OVERNIGHT. DRINK UP TO 1 QUART DAILY FOR BEST RESULTS.

HERBS/REMEDIES: SUPPORTS MILK PRODUCTION, PROMOTES REST, SUPPORTS UTERINE TONE, FOR EMOTIONAL SWINGS

TINCTURE:
- 1 PART MOTHERWORT
- 1 PART CATNIP
- ½ PART SHATAVARI
- ¼ PART CINNAMON
- ½ PART FENUGREEK* OR FENNEL

FOLLOW TINCTURE INSTRUCTIONS IN THE HERBAL PREPARATIONS CHAPTER.
*FENUGREEK MAY CAUSE GAS IN SOME PEOPLE AND BREASTFEEDING BABIES. IF THIS OCCURS, DISCONTINUE USE.

MASTITIS

THE BLEND COMBINES HERBS KNOWN FOR THEIR ANTI-INFLAMMATORY, ANTIBACTERIAL, AND LYMPHATIC-SUPPORTING PROPERTIES, WHILE ALSO PROMOTING OVERALL IMMUNE HEALTH.

HERBS/REMEDIES: CALENDULA SOOTHES INFLAMMATION AND SUPPORTS LYMPHATIC DRAINAGE, WHILE CLEAVERS PROMOTE LYMPHATIC FLOW AND REDUCE SWELLING. RED CLOVER ACTS AS AN ANTI-INFLAMMATORY, AIDING DETOXIFICATION, AND GINGER PROVIDES WARMTH, IMPROVES CIRCULATION, AND HELPS RELIEVE PAIN AND DISCOMFORT. TOGETHER, THESE HERBS BOOST THE IMMUNE SYSTEM AND HELP FIGHT OFF INFECTIONS.

TEA
- 1 PART ECHINACEA ROOT OR LEAF
- 1 PART CALENDULA FLOWERS
- 1 PART CLEAVERS
- 1 PART RED CLOVER BLOSSOMS
- ½ PART GINGER ROOT (FRESH OR DRIED)

SWEETEN TO TASTE, AND ENJOY HOT OR COLD. MAY HAVE UP TO 4 CUPS DAILY.

MASTITIS

ECHINACEA SUPPORTS THE IMMUNE SYSTEM AND HELPS COMBAT INFECTIONS.

HERBS/REMEDIES: PROVIDES EFFECTIVE SUPPORT FOR THE IMMUNE SYSTEM DURING ILLNESS.
TINCTURE

TAKE ECHINACEA TINCTURE EVERY 2-4 HOURS CONTINUE WHILE SYMPTOMS LAST AND 24 HOURS AFTER SYMPTOMS GO AWAY

HOMEOPATHY:
PHYTOLACCA DECANDRA (POKE ROOT)
HELP WITH SYMPTOMS OF MASTITIS, PARTICULARLY WHEN THE BREASTS ARE HARD, SWOLLEN, AND PAINFUL, WITH SHOOTING PAINS THAT MAY EXTEND TO OTHER PARTS OF THE BODY.
IT IS ESPECIALLY HELPFUL WHEN THERE ARE NODULES OR LUMPS IN THE BREAST, AND WHEN THE PAIN WORSENS WITH NURSING.

HERBS/REMEDIES: FOR MASTITIS, PHYTOLACCA DECANDRA IS USUALLY TAKEN IN A LOW POTENCY, SUCH AS 6C* OR 30C*, A FEW TIMES A DAY UNTIL SYMPTOMS IMPROVE.

1:100. HERE'S WHAT THE NUMBER AND "C" MEAN:
- 6C: THIS INDICATES THAT THE ORIGINAL SUBSTANCE HAS BEEN DILUTED 1 PART SUBSTANCE TO 99 PARTS WATER OR ALCOHOL, AND THEN THAT SOLUTION IS DILUTED AGAIN IN THE SAME 1:100 RATIO, REPEATED SIX TIMES.
- 30C: THIS INDICATES THAT THE ORIGINAL SUBSTANCE HAS BEEN DILUTED IN THE 1:100 RATIO THIRTY TIMES.

THE HIGHER THE NUMBER BEFORE "C," THE MORE DILUTED THE SUBSTANCE IS. IN HOMEOPATHY, IT'S BELIEVED THAT HIGHER DILUTIONS (LIKE 30C) MAY HAVE STRONGER OR LONGER-LASTING EFFECTS, DESPITE CONTAINING VERY LITTLE OR NO DETECTABLE TRACE OF THE ORIGINAL SUBSTANCE.
LOWER POTENCIES, LIKE 6C, ARE OFTEN USED FOR MORE ACUTE SYMPTOMS AND MORE FREQUENT DOSING, WHILE HIGHER POTENCIES, LIKE 30C, MAY BE USED FOR LONGER-TERM ISSUES OR LESS FREQUENT DOSING.

COMPRESS
THIS COMPRESS BLEND IS DESIGNED TO REDUCE INFLAMMATION, SUPPORT LYMPHATIC DRAINAGE, AND PROMOTE TISSUE REPAIR, OFFERING RELIEF FROM THE DISCOMFORT ASSOCIATED WITH MASTITIS.

HERBS/REMEDIES: COMFREY SOOTHES AND PROMOTES TISSUE REPAIR, WHILE MULLEIN REDUCES SWELLING WITH ITS ANTI-INFLAMMATORY PROPERTIES. CLEAVERS SUPPORT LYMPHATIC DRAINAGE, WITCH HAZEL HELPS REDUCE INFLAMMATION WITH ITS ASTRINGENT QUALITIES, AND YARROW IMPROVES CIRCULATION AND RELIEVES PAIN.

- 1 PART COMFREY LEAVES
- ½ PART MULLIEN LEAVES
- ½ PART CLEAVERS
- ½ PART WITCH HAZEL
- ½ PART YARROW

STEEP THE HERBS IN HOT WATER, LET THEM COOL SLIGHTLY, THEN SOAK A CLEAN CLOTH IN THE INFUSION. APPLY THE CLOTH TO THE AFFECTED AREA UNTIL IT COOLS (AROUND 15-20 MINUTES), REPEATING AS NEEDED.

NIPPLE HEALTH

NIPPLE BALM CRAFTED TO SOOTHE AND HEAL CRACKED OR BLEEDING NIPPLES.

HERBS/REMEDIES: SHEA BUTTER DEEPLY MOISTURIZES AND REPAIRS SKIN, COCONUT OIL HYDRATES AND OFFERS NATURAL ANTIBACTERIAL PROPERTIES, AND CALENDULA OIL SOOTHES IRRITATION AND SUPPORTS HEALING.

NIPPLE BALM:
- ½ CUP SHEA BUTTER
- ¼ CUP COCONUT OIL
- ¼ CUP CALENDULA OIL

INFUSE ¼ CUP OF CALENDULA FLOWERS INTO ½ CUP OF COCONUT OIL. STRAIN AND ADD MELTED SHEA BUTTER. POUR INTO SMALL TINS OR A SMALL JARS. AND LET COOL.

THRUSH

THESE REMEDIES CAN BE PART OF A COMPREHENSIVE APPROACH TO MANAGING THRUSH, WHICH MAY ALSO INCLUDE ANTIFUNGAL TREATMENTS PRESCRIBED BY A HEALTHCARE PROFESSIONAL.

FOR THRUSH ON THE NIPPLE:
COCONUT OIL: KNOWN FOR ITS ANTIFUNGAL PROPERTIES, COCONUT OIL CAN BE APPLIED DIRECTLY TO THE AFFECTED NIPPLES TO HELP REDUCE FUNGAL GROWTH.

TEA TREE OIL: THIS ESSENTIAL OIL HAS STRONG ANTIFUNGAL PROPERTIES. DILUTE 1-2 DROPS IN A CARRIER OIL LIKE COCONUT OIL BEFORE APPLYING TO THE NIPPLES.

CALENDULA: CALENDULA OINTMENT CAN SOOTHE IRRITATED SKIN AND HAS ANTIFUNGAL PROPERTIES THAT MAY HELP WITH NIPPLE THRUSH.

GRAPEFRUIT SEED EXTRACT: KNOWN FOR ITS ANTIFUNGAL EFFECTS, THIS EXTRACT CAN BE DILUTED AND APPLIED TO THE AFFECTED AREA.

YOGURT : APPLYING PLAIN, UNSWEETENED YOGURT DIRECTLY TO THE NIPPLES CAN HELP BALANCE THE YEAST LEVELS DUE TO ITS PROBIOTIC CONTENT.

FOR THRUSH IN A BABY'S MOUTH:
CHAMOMILE (MATRICARIA CHAMOMILLA): A CHAMOMILE TEA RINSE CAN SOOTHE THE BABY'S MOUTH AND MAY HAVE MILD ANTIFUNGAL EFFECTS.

COCONUT OIL (COCOS NUCIFERA): A SMALL AMOUNT CAN BE APPLIED TO THE BABY'S MOUTH USING A CLEAN FINGER
TO HELP REDUCE FUNGAL GROWTH.

CLOVE OIL (SYZYGIUM AROMATICUM): CLOVE OIL HAS ANTIFUNGAL PROPERTIES BUT SHOULD BE USED WITH CAUTION.
DILUTE IT IN A CARRIER OIL AND USE SPARINGLY.

NEEM (AZADIRACHTA INDICA): NEEM HAS ANTIFUNGAL PROPERTIES. A DILUTED NEEM TEA RINSE CAN BE USED TO HELP SOOTHE AND TREAT THRUSH.

PROBIOTIC YOGURT (LACTOBACILLUS ACIDOPHILUS): SWABBING A SMALL AMOUNT OF PLAIN YOGURT IN THE BABY'S
MOUTH CAN HELP RESTORE A HEALTHY BALANCE OF BACTERIA.

HYGIENE: MAINTAIN GOOD HYGIENE AND CLEAN ANY ITEMS THAT COME INTO CONTACT WITH THE AFFECTED AREAS TO PREVENT REINFECTION

TINCTURE:
SWAB BABY'S MOUTH WITH BLACK WALNUT TINCTURE (NOT TEA) DO NOT DOUBLE DIP THE COTTON SWAB.

WEANING

THESE HERBS CAN BE PART OF A HOLISTIC APPROACH TO SUPPORTING THE WEANING PROCESS, PROMOTING A DECREASE IN MILK PRODUCTION.

NETTLE (URTICA DIOICA): NETTLE CAN SUPPORT BOTH MILK PRODUCTION AND THE WEANING PROCESS. DURING WEANING, NETTLE'S NUTRIENT-RICH PROPERTIES CAN HELP NOURISH THE BODY AS IT ADJUSTS TO THE CHANGES, SUPPORTING OVERALL HEALTH AND EASING THE TRANSITION.

SAGE (SALVIA OFFICINALIS): KNOWN TO REDUCE MILK SUPPLY, SAGE CAN BE TAKEN AS A TEA (1 TSP OF DRIED SAGE PER CUP OF HOT WATER, STEEPED FOR 10 MINUTES) 2-3 TIMES DAILY. IT MAY HELP EASE THE DISCOMFORT OF ENGORGEMENT DURING WEANING.

PEPPERMINT (MENTHA PIPERITA): ANOTHER HERB THAT CAN DECREASE MILK SUPPLY, PEPPERMINT CAN BE TAKEN AS TEA OR USED IN ESSENTIAL OIL FORM (DILUTED WITH A CARRIER OIL) AND APPLIED TO THE BREASTS.

PARSLEY (PETROSELINUM CRISPUM): CONSUMING FRESH PARSLEY OR DRINKING PARSLEY TEA CAN HELP REDUCE MILK PRODUCTION.

CABBAGE LEAVES (BRASSICA OLERACEA): APPLYING TO THE BREASTS CAN REDUCE ENGORGEMENT AND EASE THE DISCOMFORT ASSOCIATED WITH WEANING. CHILL THE LEAVES BEFORE USING.

"MILK DONE" TEA
- 1 PART SAGE
- ½ PART NETTLE
- ½ PART PEPPERMINT

INFUSE 1 TBL IN CUP OF HOT WATER AND DRINK UP TO 1 QUART A DAY. STEEP FOR 10 MINUTES UP TO OVERNIGHT.

COMPRESS
- 1 PART YARROW
- ½ PART JASMINE

STEEP THE HERBS IN HOT WATER, LET THEM COOL SLIGHTLY, THEN SOAK A CLEAN CLOTH IN THE INFUSION. APPLY THE CLOTH TO THE AFFECTED AREA UNTIL COOL (AROUND 15-20 MINUTES), REPEATING AS NEEDED.

JASMINE (JASMINUM OFFICINALE) : IN REGIONS OF SOUTH ASIA, JASMINE FLOWERS ARE APPLIED TOPICALLY TO THE BREASTS TO DECREASE MILK SUPPLY. YARROW IS KNOWN FOR ITS ASTRINGENT PROPERTIES, WHICH CAN HELP DECREASE MILK SUPPLY WHEN TAKEN AS A TEA OR APPLIED AS A COMPRESS..

"Breastfeeding is a way to reclaim our bodies, our power, and our connection to our children."

— Gladys Milton, Florida Midwife

Nursing An Herb Through
(MOTHER INGESTING AND BABY NURSING)

Under six months of age, an infant's digestive system is still developing and may not be mature enough to handle much more than breast milk or formula. Therefore, it is advisable to use only herbs that are known to be safe for lactation. The amount of the herb that passes into breast milk is not exact and depends on factors such as the herb's chemical components and their fat solubility. This practice, used for generations, allows mothers to share some of the herb's benefits with their babies without negatively affecting their delicate digestive systems. For example, a mother drinking chamomile tea can pass some of its soothing benefits to a teething or colicky baby through her breast milk. Rest assured, when using safe herbs and following guidelines, this method provides gentle support for both mother and baby.

Long-term use is intended for ongoing support and gradual benefits over time. In contrast, acute use involves consuming a smaller amount more frequently for immediate relief or short-term needs.

This standard ensures that the body receives the appropriate amount based on the duration and intensity of the issue being addressed.

INFUSION / TEA

MOTHER INGESTING AND BABY NURSING

LONG TERM USE

3-4 CUPS PER DAY

ACUTE

¼ CUP, EVERY 20-30 MINUTES

TINCTURE

MOTHER INGESTING AND BABY NURSING

LONG TERM USE

½-1 TSP (30-60 DROPS), 3-4 TIMES PER DAY

ACUTE

1/8-¼ TSP (7-15 DROPS), EVERY 20-30 MINUTES

"Our ceremonies are prayers in motion, a way to give thanks and maintain harmony with all living things."

– Blackfoot Wisdom

chapter 8

The Role of Ritual
Global Traditions in Maternal Care
Creating Your Own
Postpartum Baths
Womb Massage
Belly Binding
Sacral Steaming
Honoring the Placenta
Birth As A Susto

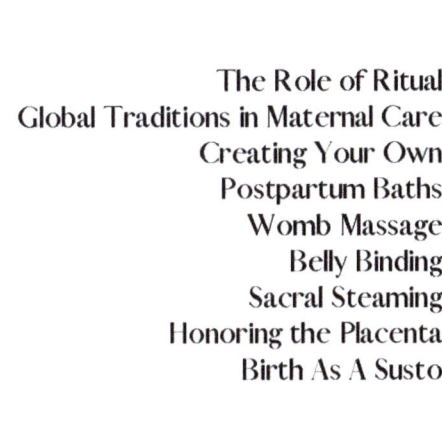

The Role of Ritual

Rituals, in their broadest sense, are actions performed with intention, often infused with meaning and purpose. They can range from the sacred and ceremonial to the everyday and mundane, with the common thread being the focus and intention behind the act. When we peak of rituals, we often think of grand ceremonies, but they can also be as simple as a daily bath or the preparation of a meal. What transforms these activities into rituals is the mindfulness and gratitude we bring to them, making them sacred acts.

In the context of pregnancy and postpartum care, rituals take on profound importance. They offer a way to honor the transformative journey of bringing new life into the world and help build a sense of community and support. Rituals provide structure, comfort, and a sense of continuity, connecting the individual to something larger than themselves—be it family, culture, or spirituality.

For instance, in many African cultures, rituals surrounding pregnancy and childbirth are deeply ingrained. The Yoruba people of Nigeria celebrate the arrival of a newborn with a naming ceremony called the *"Ikomojade,"* where the community gathers to welcome the child and offer blessings for their future. In Indigenous cultures of North America, the "Blessingway" ceremony, traditionally performed by the Navajo people, is a sacred event where a pregnant woman is surrounded by her community, who offer songs, stories, and blessings to honor her journey into motherhood.

In Latinx cultures, the *"Cuarentena"* is a postpartum ritual that involves a period of 40 days where the new mother is cared for by her community, ensuring she rests, heals, and bonds with her baby. This practice is rooted in the belief that the mother's well-being during this time is crucial for her long-term health and the health of her child.

Rituals also serve to build and strengthen communities. When people come together to celebrate life events such as graduations, baby showers, or Sweet Sixteen parties, they reinforce the bonds that hold them together. These gatherings are more than just social events; they are rituals that mark important transitions in life, providing meaning and connection.

In a holistic approach to pregnancy and postpartum care, incorporating rituals can be a powerful way to create a sense of sacredness and support. Self-care and discipline can also be ritualistic, especially during your postpartum journey. Treating yourself after birth is a ritual that honors the profound journey you've completed. Embrace small, nurturing steps like indulging in a calming herbal steam, taking a restorative bath, and applying a supportive belly wrap. Complement these practices with a soothing massage to ease tension and promote healing. These self-care rituals not only celebrate your transition into motherhood but also support your body's recovery and well-being. As Dimitris Xygalatas, a scholar of ritual studies, suggests, "Rituals help people negotiate their lives. They offer structure, comfort, and a sense of continuity. Rituals are not just relics of the past; they are essential to our mental health and social cohesion." – Dimitris Xygalatas" This perspective underscores the significance of intentional acts in the journey of motherhood, where every ritual becomes a meaningful way to honor the sacred process of bringing new life into the world.

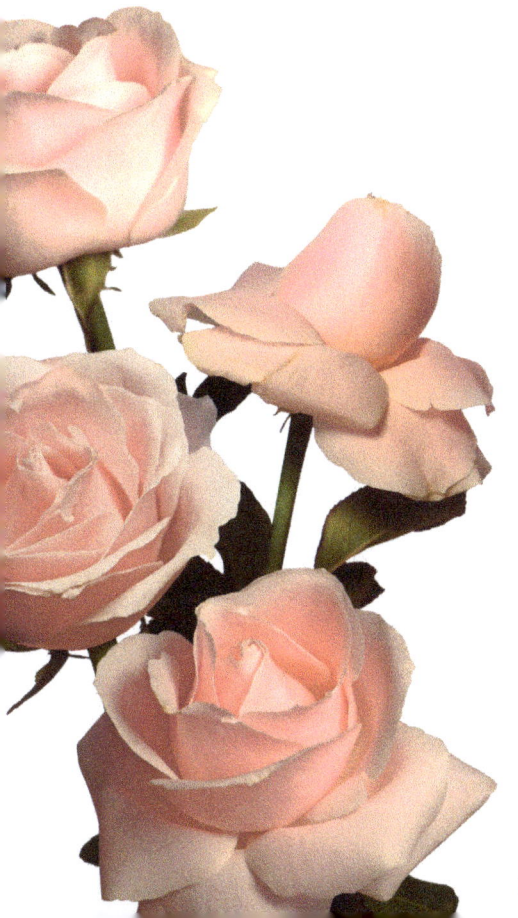

"Rituals are the language of the cosmos, the way we align ourselves with the natural order."

– Mayan Proverb

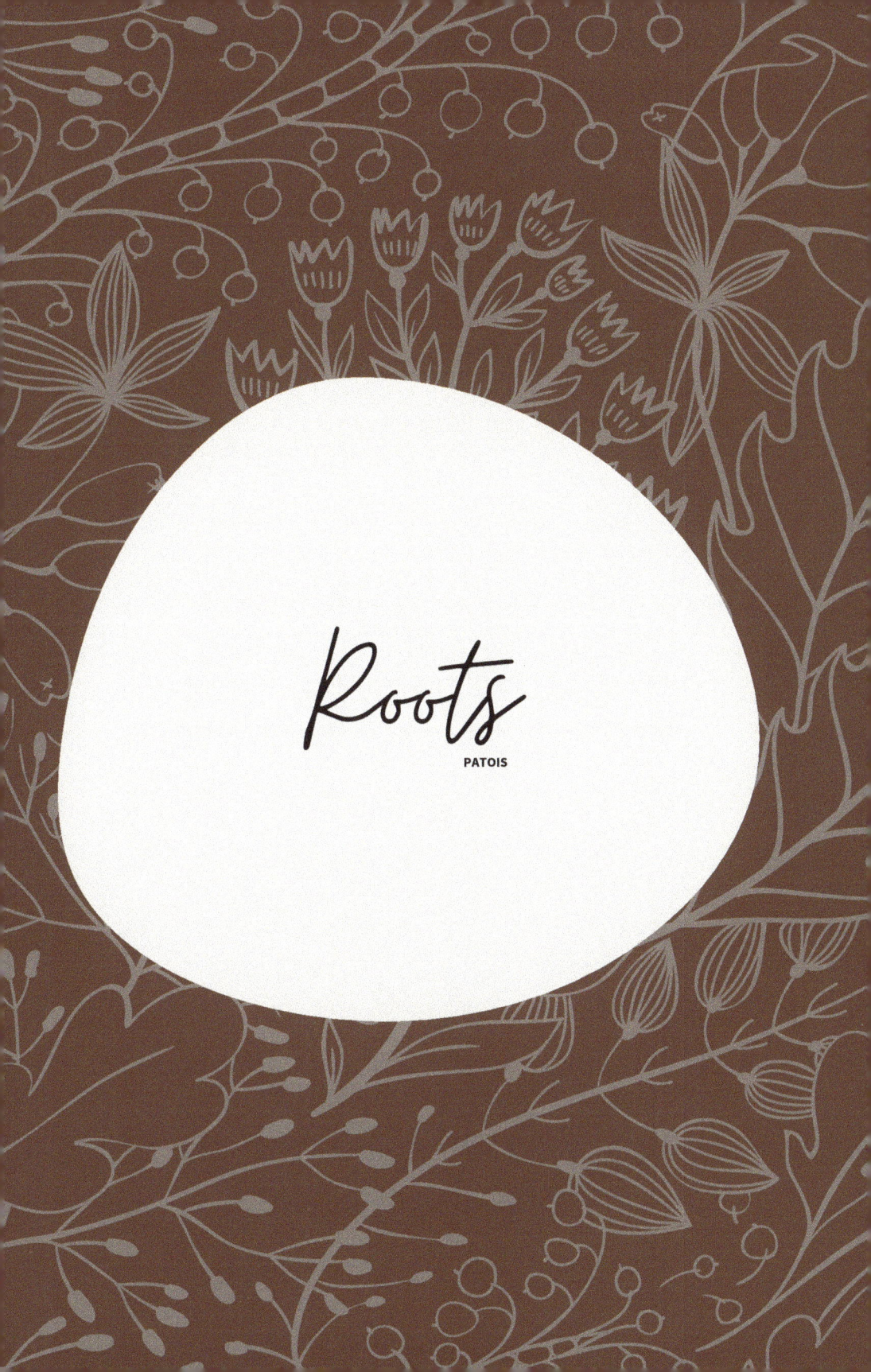

Roots
PATOIS

Guided By My Ancestors

There were things I did during my first postpartum experience that I know had to be guided by my ancestors. I stayed warm, covered my head, convalesced for a month, and felt drawn to eat and use specific herbs. This all happened before I had even researched the older ways. My first child taught me so much—most importantly, that I had no control, only the role of guiding and witnessing. I'm thankful to have learned that lesson early in my parenting journey.

For my second child, I focused on my "golden month." I had researched formulas, traditions, and foods, determined to give myself the opportunity to heal optimally. I'm so grateful for that time. I woke up and nourished myself with foods and teas, then steamed while breastfeeding and wrapped my belly. I slowly reawakened my body with lymphatic massage and stretching, doing the same for my baby. After a month of nourishment, we both emerged from our cocoon—or chrysalis, as my son recently corrected me, saying only moths come from cocoons and I should be a butterfly.

I will forever be passionate about researching plants and how they have been used over time, but I will always first honor that point of connection—that inner knowing that guided my hands as I cooked and held my baby. I am endlessly grateful for it and encourage all birthing people to embrace their inner wisdom, remembering it took thousands of years to reach you. I love my research and wanted to share some of the beautiful traditions I've witnessed or read about here.

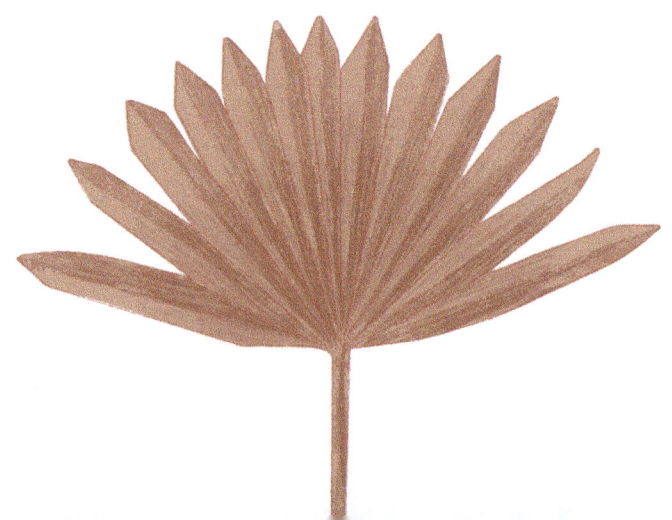

Global Traditions in Maternal Care

Indigenous Traditions (North America)

Sweat Lodge Ceremonies
Cultures: Various Indigenous tribes
Description: A purification ritual performed before childbirth to cleanse the body and spirit. It involves sitting in a steam-heated sweat lodge, where prayers and songs are offered.

Placenta Rituals
Cultures: Navajo, Cherokee, and others
Description: The placenta is treated with respect and often buried in a special place to ensure the child's connection to their homeland.

Cradleboard Making
Cultures: Various Native American tribes
Description: The creation of a cradleboard, often during pregnancy, involving prayers and blessings. The cradleboard symbolizes protection and care.

Indigenous Traditions (Central and South America)

Cuarentena (Quarantine)
Cultures: Various Indigenous cultures in Central and South America
Description: A postpartum tradition where the mother is cared for by female relatives and is restricted from certain activities for 40 days, focusing on rest, recovery, and bonding with the newborn.

Temazcal (Sweat Lodge)
Cultures: Aztec, Maya, and others
Description: Similar to the Native American sweat lodge, the temazcal is used for purification and healing. Pregnant women may participate before giving birth, and new mothers may use it postpartum for cleansing.

Manteada (Rebozo Massage)
Cultures: Various Indigenous cultures in Mexico
Description: A technique using a long scarf (rebozo) to massage the pregnant woman's abdomen, back, and hips, used to reposition the baby, relieve discomfort, and aid in labor.

Ceremonial Meal
Cultures: Various Indigenous cultures in Central and South America
Description: Special foods and drinks are prepared for the new mother, often incorporating traditional herbs and ingredients believed to aid recovery and milk production.

Aboriginal Traditions (Australia)

Birthing on Country
Cultures: Various Aboriginal Australian groups
Description: Women give birth in familiar, sacred lands, emphasizing connection to land and ancestors, promoting a sense of belonging and spiritual continuity.

Traditional Birthing Stories
Cultures: Various Aboriginal Australian groups
Description: Elders share stories and songs conveying birthing knowledge and practices, providing guidance on navigating the birthing process with ancestral wisdom.

Traditional Chinese Practices

Zuo Yuezi (Postpartum Confinement)
Cultures: Chinese
Description: A postpartum tradition where new mothers observe a month-long period of rest and recuperation, advised to avoid cold foods and focus on gentle activities to restore strength and health.

Moxibustion
Cultures: Chinese
Description: Burning mugwort (moxa) near specific acupuncture points to enhance circulation and improve overall energy, often applied during pregnancy to support fetal position and ease discomfort.

Chinese Herbal Remedies
Cultures: Chinese
Description: The use of specific herbs to support various stages of pregnancy and postpartum recovery, with formulas tailored to individual needs to address issues like energy, mood, and recovery.

African Traditions

Cultures: Various African cultures
Description: New mothers may be bathed in water infused with specific herbs to promote healing and purification. This ritual is often performed daily for a period after childbirth.

Seclusion Period
Cultures: Various West African cultures
Description: Pregnant women may be secluded during the final stages of pregnancy to ensure protection and focus on spiritual and physical preparation for childbirth. This period allows them to receive care from elder women and midwives.

Naming Ceremonies (e.g., "Outdooring")
Cultures: Akan (Ghana), Yoruba (Nigeria)
Description: A ritual to introduce the newborn to the community, often held on the seventh or eighth day after birth. The baby receives its name during this ceremony, which is filled with prayers, blessings, and offerings to ancestors and deities.

Belly Binding
Cultures: Various African cultures
Description: After birth, the mother's abdomen is wrapped tightly with cloth. This practice supports the healing process, helps the uterus shrink back to its original size, and supports the abdominal muscles.

Herbal Baths
Cultures: Various African cultures
Description: New mothers may be bathed in water infused with specific herbs to promote healing and purification. This ritual is often performed daily for a period after childbirth.

Cultures: Ancient Egyptian
Description: Amulets and charms were used to protect the mother and child during pregnancy and childbirth. These often depicted deities associated with fertility and childbirth, like Hathor and Bes.

Ceremonial Cleansing
Cultures: Ancient Egyptian
Description: Rituals involving ceremonial cleansing were performed to purify the mother before and after childbirth. This practice was believed to ensure a safe and blessed birth.

African Diaspora Traditions

Birth Songs and Drumming
Cultures: Various Afro-Caribbean and African American communities
Description: Music, singing, and drumming play an important role in the birthing process, helping to create a supportive and spiritually uplifting environment.

Ancestral Offerings
Cultures: African Diaspora, particularly in Afro-Caribbean and Brazilian traditions
Description: Offerings are made to ancestors and deities to protect the mother and child. This may include food, drink, and prayers.

Spiritual Cleansing
Cultures: Afro-Brazilian, Haitian Vodou, and others
Description: Spiritual baths and cleansing rituals may be performed for the mother and baby to protect them from negative energies and to ensure a peaceful start to the child's life.

Celtic Traditions

Brigid's Well Blessing
Cultures: Celtic
Description: A blessing performed by visiting a sacred well associated with the goddess Brigid, believed to bring fertility and protection to the mother and child.

Moon Rituals
Cultures: Celtic
Description: Celebrations and rituals aligned with lunar cycles, which are thought to influence fertility and birth. The phases of the moon are seen as having a significant impact on the natural rhythms of life.

Druid Traditions

Druidic Blessing Ceremonies
Cultures: Druidic
Description: Ceremonies performed to bless the mother and child, invoking the natural elements and deities associated with fertility and protection. These rituals often emphasize harmony with nature.

Tree Symbolism
Cultures: Druidic
Description: Trees are considered sacred in Druidic tradition, and rituals involving tree symbolism may be used to invoke strength and support for the mother and child, reflecting the interconnectedness of life.

Common Elements Across Cultures

Herbal Medicine
The use of herbal remedies to support pregnancy, labor, and postpartum recovery is a common thread in many traditions. These herbs are often chosen for their medicinal and symbolic properties.

Community Involvement
Pregnancy and childbirth are communal experiences, with family and community members actively participating in support and celebration.

Spirituality and Ancestry
Many rituals include prayers, offerings, and invocations of ancestors and deities, highlighting the spiritual dimension of childbirth.
These traditions are often passed down through generations and are integral to cultural identity. They reflect a holistic understanding of pregnancy and childbirth, blending physical care with spiritual and emotional support.

Creating Your Own

If you do not see yourself reflected in any of the listed examples, I encourage you to create your own ceremony or ritual that aligns with your personal journey, values, and cultural background. Rituals offer a profound way to honor significant life events, providing comfort, connection, and a sense of belonging. By crafting a ritual that speaks to your unique experiences, you can establish a meaningful tradition that resonates deeply with you and your community. Here are two inspirations to guide you as you design your own personal ritual, drawing from universal themes of healing, connection, and celebration:

Creating Your Own Pregnancy Circle of Support

Gathering:
Organize a gathering of the mother's closest friends and family members.

Grounding:
Begin with a grounding exercise, such as deep breathing or a short meditation. I suggest the opening meditation in this book that connects you to all the mothers and grandmothers before you.

Sharing:
Each participant shares a story, advice, or a personal experience related to pregnancy or motherhood.

Ritual:
Engage in a symbolic act, such as braiding yarn or string to represent the interconnectedness of the circle. This can be accompanied by symbolic gestures, such as tying a string around each participant's wrist to create a "bracelet of support" for the mother. In Ecuador, women stand in a circle around the mother-to-be, wrapping a long string around their wrists, connecting to the other women and the mother-to-be. She is honored and showered with flowers, and each string is cut and tied into a bracelet, worn until the baby arrives to keep the baby in the community's thoughts and prayers.

Gift:
The mother can receive a special piece of jewelry or an item that symbolizes the circle's support.

Conclusion:
Conclude with a group affirmation or a shared song, reinforcing the mother's strength and resilience.

Creating Your Own Postpartum Ritual

1. Gather the Community
- Invitation: When the mother is ready to receive visitors or leave her rest period, invite close friends, family, and other supportive women from the community.
- Location: The gathering can take place at the mother's home, a community center, or a peaceful outdoor location.
2. Create a Sacred Space
- Seating: Arrange seating in a circle to symbolize unity and equality.
- Altar: Consider adding elements like a small altar with items that hold significance for the mother.
3. Opening Ceremony
- Grounding: Begin with a grounding activity, such as meditation, a group prayer, or a moment of silence to center everyone in the space.
- Welcome: Greet everyone and express the purpose of the gathering.
4. Share Blessings and Wisdom
- Offerings: Each participant can take turns offering blessings, positive affirmations, or words of wisdom to the new mother.
- Stories: Participants may also share personal stories of motherhood, offering advice or support.
5. Gift Giving:
- Individual Gifts: The community can offer small, meaningful gifts to the mother, such as handmade items, letters, or something that represents love and care.
- Communal Gift: A communal gift, like a postpartum care package with teas, herbs, and comfort items, could also be prepared.
6. Nourish the Body
- Meal Sharing: Share a meal or light refreshments prepared by the community, including traditional postpartum foods that are nourishing and healing. This act reinforces the sense of community and care.
7. Closing Ceremony
- Candle Ritual: End the circle with a closing ritual, such as lighting a candle that the mother can take home, symbolizing the ongoing support of the community.
- Group Activity:
- Group singing, chanting, or a collective "thank you" can create a powerful conclusion to the ceremony.
8. Follow-Up Support:
- Ongoing Support: Encourage the community to continue supporting the mother through postpartum visits, meals, or helping with childcare.
- Support Network: Establish a postpartum support network where the mother can reach out if she needs assistance or companionship.

"In our culture, rituals are not just traditions; they are acts of love that bind us to our roots and to each other."

— Sandra Cisneros

Postpartum Baths

Herbal postpartum baths hold deep significance across various cultures, intertwining spirituality, tradition, and medicinal benefits into a holistic practice of healing and renewal. These baths go beyond mere hygiene; they are a sacred ritual that honors the journey of childbirth, supports recovery, and fosters a profound connection between the mother and her new role.

In many traditions, herbal postpartum baths are a cornerstone of postpartum care, imbued with spiritual meaning. For instance, in Mexico and Central America, *"baños de hierbas"* are taken to cleanse and revitalize the body and spirit after childbirth. In Southeast Asia, particularly Indonesia and Malaysia, the "jamu" practice involves bathing with herbal infusions to restore the body's natural balance. Similarly, in the Himalayan region, postpartum bathing rituals using herbs like neem and turmeric purify and rejuvenate, often accompanied by meditation or chanting to enhance the spiritual experience.

Medicinally, these baths offer a range of benefits. The combination of warm water and therapeutic herbs aid tissue repair, reduce perineal soreness, and alleviate discomfort. Anti-inflammatory herbs such as calendula and chamomile soothe the body, while rosemary and nettle stimulate blood flow, aiding in the reduction of postpartum bleeding. Calming herbs like lavender and rose petals promote relaxation, helping new mothers manage stress and improve sleep. Additionally, herbs with antimicrobial properties, like witch hazel and sage, support vaginal health and help prevent infections.

Symbolically, herbal postpartum baths represent the transition from pregnancy to motherhood, offering a time for self-care and reflection. This practice allows mothers to connect deeply with their bodies, enhancing emotional well-being and providing a moment of tranquility during the busy postpartum period.

While bathing during pregnancy also offers benefits—such as easing muscle tension and improving circulation—it is important to note that warm baths, rather than hot, are recommended, and some herbs should be avoided during pregnancy.

For those who prefer modern conveniences, pre-made herbal bath soaks and infusions offer similar benefits, making it easier to integrate this healing practice into contemporary postpartum care.

In essence, herbal postpartum baths are a powerful blend of spiritual, traditional, and medicinal practices. By embracing these rituals, new mothers can honor their journey, support their healing, and connect deeply with the transformative experience of motherhood.

POSTPARTUM BATHS

HERBAL BATHS IN THE POSTPARTUM PERIOD CAN PROVIDE BOTH PHYSICAL AND MENTAL BENEFITS, PROMOTING HEALING AND RELAXATION. PHYSICALLY, THEY CAN HELP SOOTHE SORE MUSCLES, REDUCE INFLAMMATION, AND SUPPORT UTERINE RECOVERY, WHILE MENTALLY, THE CALMING AROMAS AND WARM WATER CAN ALLEVIATE STRESS, ENHANCE MOOD, AND ENCOURAGE A SENSE OF CONNECTION WITH ONESELF AND THE NEW BABY

INSTRUCTIONS:
BRING WATER TO A BOIL AND THEN SIMMER THE HERBS TOGETHER IN A LARGE POT OF WATER ON FOR 20-30 MINUTES.
STRAIN THE MIXTURE AND ADD IT TO A WARM BATH.
SOAK FOR AT LEAST 20 MINUTES, ALLOWING THE WARMTH AND HERBS TO SOOTHE AND HEAL

HERBS/REMEDIES:

1. AVOCADO: RICH IN ANTIOXIDANTS, AVOCADO LEAVES HELP TO SOOTHE THE SKIN AND REDUCE INFLAMMATION. THEY ARE ALSO BELIEVED TO SUPPORT POSTPARTUM HEALING.
2. RUE (RUDA): TRADITIONALLY USED TO STIMULATE CIRCULATION, RELIEVE PAIN, AND PROVIDE EMOTIONAL BALANCE.
3. YARROW: KNOWN FOR ITS ASTRINGENT PROPERTIES, YARROW HELPS TO TONE AND HEAL THE SKIN, AS WELL AS REDUCE BLEEDING.
4. ROSE: ADDED FOR THEIR CALMING AND UPLIFTING EFFECTS, ROSE PETALS ALSO PROMOTE SKIN HEALING AND EMOTIONAL WELL-BEING.
5. GUINEA HEN WEED (ANAMU): USED FOR ITS ANTIMICROBIAL PROPERTIES, IT HELPS PREVENT INFECTIONS.
6. BAY LEAVES: TRADITIONALLY USED TO IMPROVE CIRCULATION AND REDUCE MUSCLE TENSION.
7. CINNAMON STICKS: ADDED FOR WARMTH AND TO STIMULATE CIRCULATION.
8. MANGO LEAVES: SOOTHE SKIN IRRITATIONS, TREAT BURNS, REDUCE INFLAMMATION, AND PROVIDE ANTIMICROBIAL PROTECTION FOR MINOR WOUNDS AND INFECTIONS.
9. ROSEMARY (ROMERO): HELPS TO RELAX MUSCLES AND PROMOTE MENTAL CLARITY.
10. LAVENDER: ADDED FOR ITS CALMING PROPERTIES, WHICH CAN HELP REDUCE STRESS AND PROMOTE RELAXATION
11. KATRAFAY: USED FOR ITS STRONG ANTI-INFLAMMATORY EFFECTS AND TO SOOTHE ACHING MUSCLES.
12. SHEA LEAVES: KNOWN FOR THEIR MOISTURIZING AND SKIN-HEALING PROPERTIES.
13. LEMONGRASS: USED FOR ITS REFRESHING SCENT AND TO HELP REDUCE POSTPARTUM FATIGUE.
14. GINGER PEEL (SHENG JIANG PI): WARMING AND PROMOTES CIRCULATION, REDUCES SWELLING, AND SUPPORTS POSTPARTUM RECOVERY.
15. MUGWORT (AI YE): STIMULATES BLOOD CIRCULATION, ALLEVIATES PAIN, AND SUPPORTS UTERINE HEALTH WITH ITS WARMING PROPERTIES.
16. RAMULUS CINNAMOMI (CINNAMON TWIG): WARMS CHANNELS AND PROMOTES CIRCULATION, CRUCIAL FOR POSTPARTUM RECOVERY.
17. DIVARICATE SAPOSHNIKOVIA (FANG FENG OR SILVER ROOT): EXPELS WIND AND DAMPNESS, PROVIDING RELIEF FROM POSTPARTUM ACHES AND PAINS.
18. TETRADIUM RUTICARPUM (EVODIA FRUIT, WU ZHU YU): WARMING AND PAIN-RELIEVING
19. COMFREY LEAF: PROMOTES SKIN HEALING AND REDUCES INFLAMMATION, SOOTHING POSTPARTUM SORENESS.
20. CALENDULA: CALMS AND HEALS IRRITATED OR SENSITIVE SKIN.
21. MYRRH POWDER: ANTISEPTIC PROPERTIES PREVENT INFECTION AND SUPPORT HEALING.
22. BAKING SODA: NEUTRALIZES SKIN ACIDITY AND SOOTHES IRRITATION.
23. EPSOM SALT (PER BATH): RELAXES MUSCLES, REDUCES SWELLING, AND PROMOTES HEALING.

Herbal Baths

POSTPARTUM BATHS

LYANI'S BATH
- 1 PART AVOCADO LEAVES
- ½ PART RUE (RUDA)
- 1 PART YARROW
- ½ PART ROSE BUDS

HAITIAN POSTPARTUM BATH:
- 1 PART GUINEA HEN WEED (ANAMU)
- ½ PART MANGO LEAVES
- ½ PART BAY LEAVES
- 2 CINNAMON STICKS PER BATH

MEXICAN POSTPARTUM BATH:
- 1/3 PART RUDA (RUE)
- 1/3 PART ROMERO (ROSEMARY)
- 1/3 PART LAVENDER

WEST AFRICAN BATH:
- 1 BALL OF KATRAFAY
- ½ PART SHEA LEAVES
- ½ PART LEMONGRASS

TCM GINGER BATH
- 1 PART GINGER PEEL
- 1 PART MUGWORT (AI YE)
- 1 PART RAMULUS CINNAMOMI (CINNAMON TWIG)
- 1 PART DIVARICATE SAPOSHNIKOVIA (FANG FENG OR SILVER ROOT)
- ½ PART TETRADIUM RUTICARPUM (EVODIA FRUIT, WU ZHU YU)
- 1 PART LEMONGRASS

FLORAL BATH
- 2 PARTS COMFREY LEAF
- 1 PART CALENDULA
- 1 PART LAVENDER
- ½ PART MYRRH POWDER*
- ½ PART ROSE BUDS
- ¼ PART BAKING SODA
- 1 CUP SEA SALT OR EPSOM SALT PER BATH

*A 2019 STUDY AT HAFEZ HOSPITAL IN SHIRAZ, IRAN, FOUND THAT SITZ BATHS WITH MYRRH EXTRACT WERE MORE EFFECTIVE FOR EPISIOTOMY WOUND HEALING IN PRIMIPAROUS WOMEN THAN POVIDONE IODINE, THE STANDARD TREATMENT AT THE TIME. THE RESEARCH SUGGESTS THAT MYRRH MAY ENHANCE THE PRESENCE OF FIBROBLASTS AT WOUND SITES. IN TRADITIONAL PERSIAN MEDICINE, MYRRH (COMMIPHORA MYRRHA) AND FRANKINCENSE (BOSWELLIA CARTERI) ARE COMMONLY USED BY MIDWIVES FOR TOPICAL WOUND CARE

POSTPARTUM SITZ BATHS

SITZ BATH ARE HELPFUL FOR SOOTHING INFLAMED PERINEAL TISSUE AND HEMMROHIODS AFTER CHILDBIRTH.

MIX THE HERB INTO A BLEND. ADD ¼ CUP OF HERBS TO 6 CUPS OF BOILING WATER. REMOVE FROM HEAT AND COVER AND LET STEEP FOR AT LEAST 20 MINUTES. STRAIN THE LIQUID USING A MESH STRAINER AND ADD TO BATH. ENJOY AND SOAK FOR UP TO 20 MINUTES UP TO THREE TIMES A DAY.

THIS SOOTHING BATH BLEND HAS ANTISEPTIC, ANTI-INFLAMMATORY AND VULNERARY. THIS RECIPE WORKS AS A SITZ BATH OR IT CAN BE PLACED IN A "PERIBOTTLE" USED IN SHOWER OR AFTER URINATING.

SITZ & SOOTHE .
- 1 PART CALENDULA
- 1 PART YARROW – 1 PT
- 1 PART CHAMOMILE – 1 PT
- 1 PART PLANTAIN LEAVES 1 PT
- ½ PART UVA URSI OR WITCH HAZEL LEAVES
- ½ PART LAVENDER
- ½ CUP EPSOM SALT PER SITZ BATH

"Rituals are the heartbeat of our people, a way to honor the ancestors and bring forth their wisdom."

– Yoruba Proverb

Womb Massage

Postpartum womb massage, often referred to as abdominal or "Mayan" massage, is an ancient practice deeply rooted in traditions such as those of the *K'iche', Kaqchikel, and Yucatec* peoples. For many, it is not just about physical healing; it is a profound way to reconnect with the womb, honor the postpartum journey, and restore balance within the body. In many cultures, this practice is seen as a sacred ritual essential for a mother's recovery after childbirth, supporting the body's natural processes and fostering a deep connection with the womb.

From a physiological standpoint, the massage promotes uterine health and supports the body's natural recovery process after childbirth. By stimulating circulation in the abdominal area, it helps reduce swelling and supports the involution of the uterus, the process by which the uterus shrinks back to its pre-pregnancy size. Regular massage can also aid in the expulsion of remaining lochia (postpartum discharge) and reduce the risk of uterine infections. Additionally, it can alleviate cramping and bloating by encouraging the proper alignment of the uterus, which helps prevent complications like uterine prolapse.

After childbirth, the uterus may not always return to its original position, which can lead to discomfort, prolonged bleeding, and, some cultures believe, emotional imbalance. Properly massaging the womb helps guide it back into place, supporting optimal healing and preventing complications. In Mesoamerican cultures, the womb is seen as a powerful source of feminine energy, and after childbirth, it undergoes significant changes. Womb massage is meant to help women reconnect with this vital part of their being and ground themselves in their bodies.

After childbirth, the uterus gradually shrinks and descends back into the pelvic cavity. In the first few days postpartum, the top of the uterus (fundus) should be located around the level of the belly button or slightly above. As the days progress, the uterus continues to shrink and move downward, eventually returning to its position behind the pubic bone. To gauge the position of the womb, gently press on the lower abdomen, feeling for any tenderness, firmness, or hardness. It might feel firm, like a small, rounded ball with a smooth surface. As the postpartum period progresses, it should gradually descend and become softer, resting about two to three fingers' width below the belly button.

If your womb feels off-center, lower than expected, or isn't shrinking properly, a gentle massage can help realign it. When performed correctly it is a gentle, non-invasive method to support overall reproductive health, and recovery.

While postpartum womb massage can be beneficial for many women, there are certain situations where it may be contraindicated or require extra caution. It is essential to consult with a healthcare provider before beginning any postpartum massage, especially if any of the following conditions apply:

Cesarean Section Recovery: Women who have had a cesarean section should avoid abdominal massage until their incision has fully healed. Even after healing, massage should be done with extreme care to avoid disrupting scar tissue. Always consult with a healthcare provider before starting womb massage in this case.

Infection or Fever: If there are signs of infection, such as fever, redness, or unusual discharge, womb massage should be avoided until the infection has been fully treated. Massage in these cases could potentially spread the infection or exacerbate symptoms.

Severe Postpartum Hemorrhage: Women who have experienced severe postpartum hemorrhage should avoid womb massage until they have fully recovered. This condition can make the uterus more sensitive, and massage may cause further complications.

Placenta Retention: If there is any suspicion that part of the placenta has been retained in the uterus, massage should be avoided until the situation has been medically resolved. Retained placenta can cause serious complications.

Severe Diastasis Recti: Women with severe diastasis recti (separation of the abdominal muscles) should approach womb massage with caution. In these cases, abdominal massage should be done under the guidance of a womb massage professional or physical therapist to avoid further straining the muscles.

Recent Pelvic Surgery: If a woman has had any recent pelvic or abdominal surgery unrelated to childbirth, womb massage may need to be postponed until full recovery.

Active Blood Clots: If there is a known history of blood clots, especially in the legs or lungs, womb massage may be contraindicated, as it could potentially dislodge clots and cause serious complications.

Severe Anemia or Weakness: Women who are severely anemic or extremely weak postpartum, may need to wait until their strength has returned before engaging in womb massage.

Womb Massage At Home

Create a Sacred Space: Find a quiet, comfortable space where you won't be disturbed. Light a candle, play soft music, or burn some incense to set a calming atmosphere.

Warm the Oil: Choose an oil and gently warm it by placing the bottle in a bowl of warm water for a few minutes. Herbal-infused oils can enhance the massage, offering anti-inflammatory benefits, promoting circulation, and deeply nourishing the skin and tissues. The herbs' aroma also adds a calming, grounding effect.

Lie Down Comfortably: Lie on your back with a pillow under your knees to support your lower back. Take a few deep breaths to relax.

Begin the Massage: Pour a small amount of oil into your hands and rub them together to distribute the oil evenly. Start by gently massaging your lower abdomen in a clockwise circular motion, beginning just above your pubic bone and moving towards your belly button.

Focus on Your Womb: As you massage, focus on the area where your womb is located. You can use your fingertips to gently press into the tissues, feeling for any areas of tension or tenderness. Spend extra time on areas that feel tight or uncomfortable.

Visualize Healing: As you massage, visualize your womb being bathed in healing energy. Imagine it moving back into its natural position, supported by your loving attention.

Finish with Rest: After your massage, take a few moments to rest with your hands placed over your womb. Close your eyes and breathe deeply, allowing the energy of the massage to integrate into your body.

Connecting with Your Womb: Postpartum womb massage goes beyond physical realignment; it's a way to reconnect with your womb on a deeper level. After childbirth, the womb often feels overlooked as focus shifts to the newborn. This practice allows you to honor its importance and the incredible journey it has undergone.

This practice also serves as a meditative moment, a time to reflect on your postpartum journey and the new life you have brought into the world. It allows you to tune into your body's needs, fostering a sense of empowerment and self-awareness. This ancient ritual is a beautiful way to honor your journey into motherhood, supporting your body's natural healing processes and fostering a sense of peace and well-being.

"Belly binding is not just about aesthetics or bouncing back. It's a centuries-old practice rooted in cultures that understand the profound shift that occurs in a birthing person's body. Wrapping is a way of supporting the healing process, both physically and emotionally, and it's a form of care that acknowledges the intense work a body has done in bringing forth new life."

Angelique Geehan, a doula and birth worker

Support Over Snapback

"Belly casing" is a cultural practice of wrapping the abdomen, especially after childbirth, to support the abdominal muscles and organs as they return to their pre-pregnancy state. Known by various names across different cultures, this practice has deep historical roots and is often tied to traditional postpartum care aimed at aiding recovery and restoring the body's natural balance.

Terms for belly binding vary around the world, including *"faja"* in Latin America, *"bengkung"* in Malaysia and Indonesia, *"sarashi"* in Japan, "tying the stomach" in Jamaica, "wrapping the belly" in various African cultures, *"le binding"* in Haiti, *"tapal"* in the Philippines, and "girdle" or "shapewear" in modern Western contexts.

The purpose of belly wrapping is to provide gentle compression and support, not to force a return to a pre-pregnancy body shape. Its primary goal is to assist the uterus in contracting back to its original size and offer stability as the abdominal muscles and tissues heal after childbirth. This support can help new mothers feel more secure and comfortable during their postpartum recovery.

The pressure to quickly revert to a pre-pregnancy body can be both physically and mentally damaging. Unrealistic standards can create unnecessary stress and detract from the focus on recovery and self-care. When approached with the right mindset, belly binding can honor and support the body's natural healing process rather than conform to external expectations. Emphasizing recovery over aesthetics can combat harmful standards and promote a healthier, more compassionate postpartum experience.

Belly wrapping offers numerous benefits, including abdominal support, improved posture, and reduced postpartum bleeding. While traditional methods may not suit everyone, modern belly wraps and compression garments provide similar advantages in a more convenient form. Although many cultures moved away from belly wrapping due to shifts in postpartum care, it is now experiencing a resurgence as interest in holistic and traditional practices grows. This revival reflects a desire for nurturing ways to honor the postpartum journey.

In summary, belly casing is a practice deeply rooted in many cultures, providing valuable support and care. The core belief remains that supporting the abdomen during postpartum aids physical recovery and can complement other nurturing rituals that emphasize community support and holistic well-being.

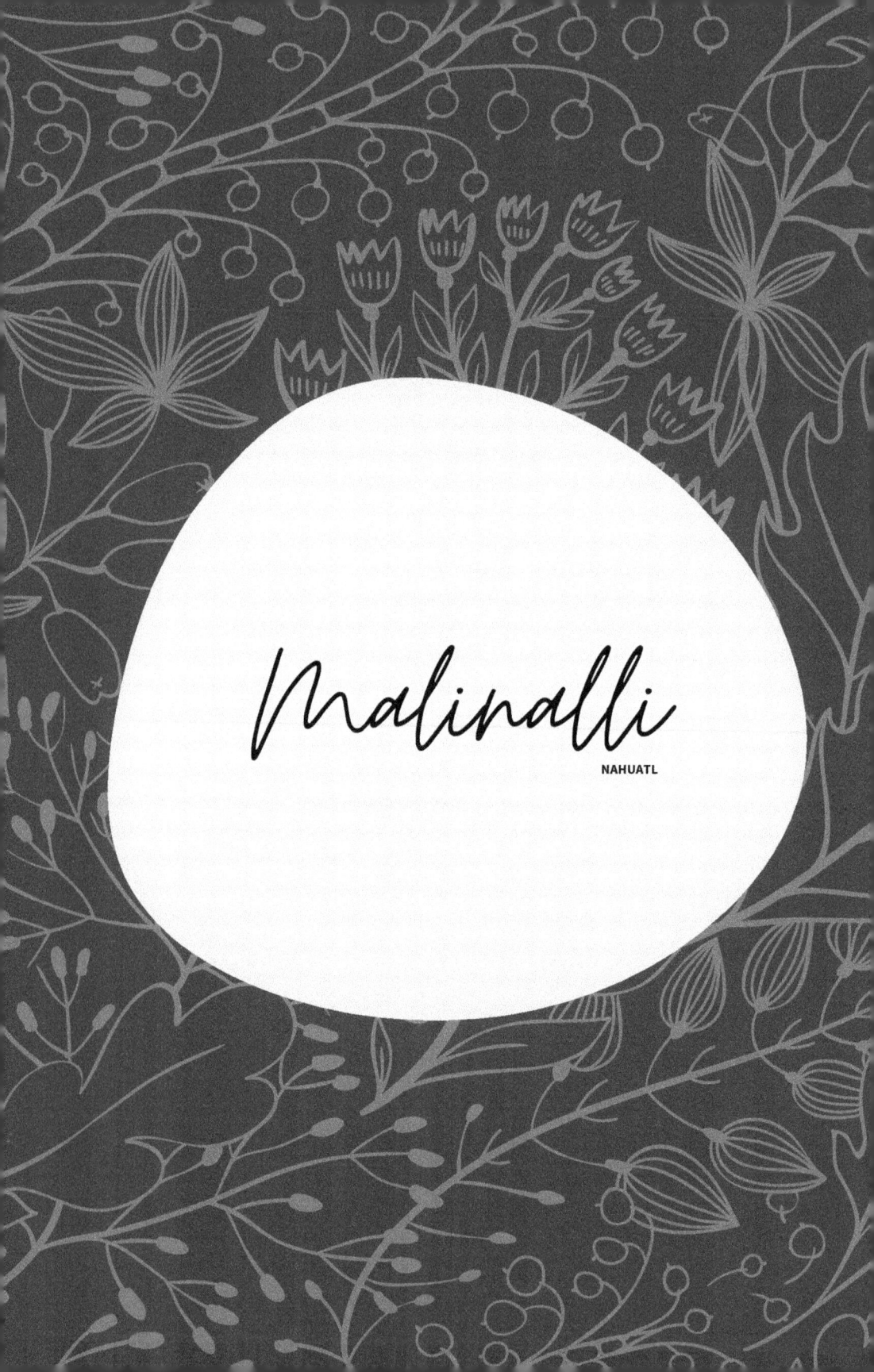

Sacral Steaming

Sacral steaming, also known as Peristeam Hydrotherapy, is a practice where an individual sits or squats over steaming water infused with medicinal herbs. It is more than just a physical practice—it is a deeply ritualistic act of self-care that offers both physiological and psychological benefits. This tradition, deeply rooted in cultures across Africa, Asia, Central America, and some European countries, has been used for centuries as part of postpartum recovery to support new mothers in their healing journey.

One of the profound psychological benefits of sacral steaming is its ability to boost oxytocin levels, the hormone often referred to as the "love hormone." This increase in oxytocin not only enhances feelings of bonding and emotional well-being but also plays a critical role in aiding milk let-down, making breastfeeding smoother for the new mother. The warmth and herbal steam work synergistically to increase circulation to the pelvic area, which can help to bring comfort and support the body's natural healing processes.

However, the most powerful aspect of sacral steaming lies in its role as a ritual of self-care. In the midst of the demands of new motherhood, this practice offers a dedicated pause—a moment to focus on oneself, to nurture the body, and to honor the transformative journey of childbirth. With each session, the intention to heal and care for oneself is reaffirmed, making sacral steaming not just a physical therapy, but a holistic ritual that encompasses both body and spirit.

The concept that steaming is used to "clean" the vagina can be problematic and rooted in a patriarchal view that the functions of women's bodies are dirty. The vagina does not need to be "cleaned" and although steam is considered cleansing it should be viewed more as a transdermal delivery of herbs into the skin and then blood stream. It encourages circulation directly to the area that requires care.

Although sacral steaming is deeply rooted in tradition and has seen a resurgence in popularity, it continues to be a topic of debate among health professionals. Some view its benefits as being more culturally significant than based on physiological effects. However, small clinical studies, such as those conducted by Steamy Chick, have shown promising results for postpartum sacral steaming.

These studies suggest that this ritual may offer several benefits during postpartum recovery, including:

- Lowering blood pressure and pulse: The warmth of the steam, combined with the healing properties of herbs, promotes relaxation and circulatory health.
- Uterine restoration: Sacral steaming may assist in the uterus returning to its pre-pregnancy size.
- Waist girth and weight loss: The practice has been associated with a quicker reduction in waist size and overall weight.
- Labia healing: The soothing warmth of the steam can aid in the healing of the labia.
- Quicker cessation of uterine bleeding: Steaming can help draw out lochia, potentially speeding up the end of postpartum bleeding.
- Alleviating suture discomfort: The warmth may help ease discomfort from any stitches.
- Promoting bowel regularity and hemorrhoid reduction: The steam can stimulate bowel movements and reduce hemorrhoid swelling.
- It is possible that steaming positively impacts other postpartum indicators such as breast milk supply, preeclampsia prevention or treatment, incontinence prevention and promotion of urination.

While these initial findings are encouraging, exploring them further through larger sample sizes and additional studies could provide deeper insights and strengthen our understanding.

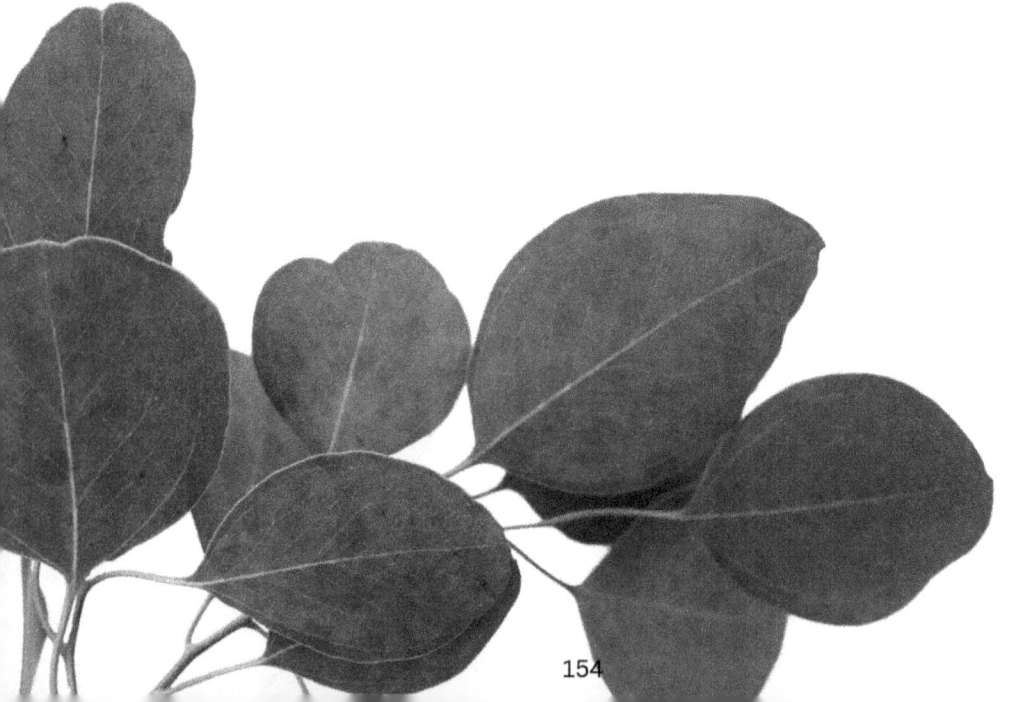

SETTING UP THE STEAM

PREPARE THE AREA:
CREATE A CALM, COMFORTABLE SPACE WHERE YOU CAN SIT OR SQUAT SAFELY. ENSURE THE AREA IS CLEAN, AND HAVE ALL YOUR SUPPLIES READY, INCLUDING THE HERBS, STEAMING STOOL OR CHAIR (WITH A HOLE IN THE MIDDLE), A LARGE BOWL OR POT FOR THE STEAM, AND BLANKETS OR TOWELS.

ENSURE THE ROOM IS WARM AND FREE OF DRAFTS TO PREVENT COOLING DOWN TOO QUICKLY AFTER THE STEAM.

PREPARE THE STEAM:
BOIL 2-3 QUARTS OF WATER AND POUR IT INTO A LARGE BOWL OR POT.
ADD YOUR CHOSEN HERBS (SEE HERBAL SUGGESTIONS BELOW). USE ABOUT A HANDFUL OF DRIED HERBS (APPROXIMATELY 1 CUP) OR TWICE AS MUCH FRESH HERBS.

ALLOW THE HERBS TO STEEP FOR ABOUT 5-10 MINUTES, COVERED, TO RELEASE THEIR ESSENTIAL OILS AND MEDICINAL PROPERTIES.

CHECK THE TEMPERATURE OF THE STEAM BY HOVERING YOUR HAND OVER THE BOWL.
THE STEAM SHOULD BE WARM, NOT TOO HOT, TO AVOID BURNS.

POSITIONING

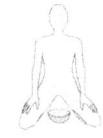
PLACE THE STEAMING BOWL OR POT UNDER A SPECIALLY DESIGNED STEAMING STOOL OR A STURDY CHAIR WITH AN OPEN SEAT.

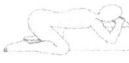
SIT OR SQUAT OVER THE STEAM, ENSURING THAT THE STEAM CAN RISE DIRECTLY TO YOUR PERINEAL AREA.
WRAP A BLANKET OR TOWEL AROUND YOUR WAIST TO KEEP THE STEAM CONTAINED AND PREVENT HEAT LOSS.

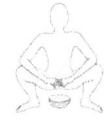
SIT FOR 10-15 MINUTES, TAKING DEEP BREATHS AND RELAXING.

RECOVERY

AFTER STEAMING, REST FOR A FEW MINUTES BEFORE GETTING UP. DRY OFF GENTLY WITH A CLEAN TOWEL.

DRESS WARMLY TO MAINTAIN BODY HEAT AND REST IN A COMFORTABLE POSITION.

CLEAN UP: DISPOSE OF THE HERBS AND THOROUGHLY CLEAN YOUR POT AFTER EACH USE.

STEAMING TO REGULATE LABOR CONTRACTIONS

STEAMING DURING LABOR CAN HELP REGULATE CONTRACTIONS BY USING THE WARMTH AND THERAPEUTIC PROPERTIES OF HERBS. THIS PRACTICE IS TYPICALLY EMPLOYED IN THE EARLY STAGES OF LABOR TO MANAGE IRREGULAR OR MILD CONTRACTIONS, PROMOTING RELAXATION. IT IS IMPORTANT TO AVOID STEAMING IF YOUR WATER HAS BROKEN OR IF THERE IS ANY SIGN OF INFECTION.

WHEN TO STEAM:
TIMING: EARLY LABOR, WHEN CONTRACTIONS ARE IRREGULAR OR MILD.
FREQUENCY: ONCE OR TWICE FOR 10-15 MINUTES. IF LABOR PROGRESSES QUICKLY, STEAMING MAY NOT BE NEEDED.

BENEFITS FOR LABOR CONTRACTIONS:
ENCOURAGING REGULAR CONTRACTIONS: THE WARMTH RELAXES PELVIC MUSCLES, FOSTERING CONSISTENT CONTRACTIONS.

RELIEVING TENSION:
STEAM EASES TENSION IN THE PERINEAL AREA, ENHANCING CONTRACTION EFFECTIVENESS.

PROMOTING CIRCULATION:
INCREASED BLOOD FLOW SUPPORTS UTERINE CONTRACTIONS AND NOURISHES TISSUES.

SAFETY CONSIDERATIONS:
AVOID STEAMING IF WATER HAS BROKEN: INCREASES INFECTION RISK.
TEMPERATURE: KEEP STEAM WARM, NOT HOT, TO PREVENT BURNS.

DURATION:
LIMIT TO 10-15 MINUTES; STOP IF FEELING LIGHTHEADED OR UNCOMFORTABLE.

HERBAL QUALITY:
USE ONLY ORGANIC OR SAFELY WILDCRAFTED HERBS.

POSTPARTUM STEAMING REGIMEN

POSTPARTUM VAGINAL STEAMS SHOULD BE VERY GENTLE. IF SITTING IS UNCOMFORTABLE OR THERE ARE STITCHES PRESENT, START WITH A FIVE-MINUTE VAGINAL STEAM, AND INCREASE TIME BY TWO OR THREE MINUTES PER DAY.

STEAMING CAN BEGIN AS SOON AS POSTPARTUM BLEEDING HAS BEGUN TO DISCERNIBLY DECREASE. FOR SOME, THAT MAY BE THE SAME DAY AND FOR OTHERS IT MAY BE A FEW DAYS.

STEAMING CAN BE RELAXING AND IS PREFERABLY DONE AT NIGHT OR BEFORE A NAP.

CONTINUE USE FOR FORTY DAYS, PREFERABLY BEFORE GOING TO BED AT NIGHT.

USE ONCE A MONTH TO ONCE EVERY THREE MONTHS FOR 15-30 MINUTES FOR MAINTENANCE THEREAFTER.

HERBS FOR STEAMING

WHEN SELECTING HERBS FOR A SACRAL STEAM, FOCUS ON THOSE THAT SUPPORT RELAXATION, CIRCULATION, ANTIMICROBIAL ACTION, ASTRINGENCY, AND UTERINE HEALTH. CHOOSING ORGANIC AND WELL-SOURCED HERBS IS ESSENTIAL TO ENSURE PURITY AND AVOID EXPOSURE TO PESTICIDES OR CONTAMINANTS. HIGH-QUALITY, ETHICALLY SOURCED HERBS IMPROVE THE SAFETY AND EFFECTIVENESS OF YOUR STEAM, PROVIDING A MORE BENEFICIAL AND SOOTHING EXPERIENCE. DIFFERENT PRACTITIONERS AND CULTURES USE THE PLANT MEDICINE THAT GROWS AROUND THEM. I ENCOURAGE READERS TO RESEARCH WHICH HERBS HAVE BEEN USED IN THEIR AREA THAT HAVE STYTPIC, ANTIMICROBIAL, AND ANIT-INFLAMMATORY PROPERTIES.

LABOR STEAM RECIPE

BENEFITS: RED RASPBERRY LEAVES SUPPORT UTERINE TONE AND EASE CONTRACTIONS, ROSEMARY PROMOTES CIRCULATION AND RELIEVES MUSCLE TENSION, AND CHAMOMILE OFFERS CALMING EFFECTS AND SOOTHES THE NERVOUS SYSTEM.

SOOTHING STEAM:
- 1 PART RED RASPBERRY LEAVES
- ½ PART ROSEMARY
- 1 PART CHAMOMILE

POSTPARTUM STEAM RECIPE

- 2 PARTS AVOCADO LEAVES
- 2 PARTS ROSEMARY
- 1 PART EUCALYPTUS

I GIVE HONOR TO THE STEWARDS OF INDIGENOUS WISDOM. THIS RECIPE WAS SHARED BY PANQUETZANI OF INDIGIEMAMA A MESOAMERICAN MEDICINE AND TRADITION KEEPER. THE BLEND CAN STAND ALONE OR AS A BASE FOR ADDITIONAL HERBS LIKE MUGWORT OR ROSE.

BLUSH BABY STEAM

- 2 PARTS GUAVA LEAVES
- 2 PARTS ROSE
- 1 PART WITCH HAZEL LEAVES

GOLDEN HOUR STEAM

- 1 PART WITCH HAZEL
- 1 PART CALENDULA
- 1 PART YARROW
- 1 PART PLANTAIN LEAF
- ½ PART CHAMOMILE
- ¼ PART LAVENDER
- ¼ PART SALT

SACRAL STEAMING

"Ritual is an opportunity to connect to yourself and the wisdom of your ancestors. It's the difference between surviving and thriving."

Latham Thomas
founder of Mama Glow

Steaming, Compresses, and Massage Oils

MANY HERBS USED FOR STEAMING CAN ALSO BE INFUSED INTO A LABOR OR POSTPARTUM MASSAGE OIL, OR INCORPORATED INTO A SOOTHING HERBAL COMPRESS OR REJUVENATING BATH.

Herb	Properties and Uses
ROSEMARY Rosmarinus Officinalis	ANTIBACTERIAL, TONIC, ASTRINGENT, DISINFECTANT. USED AS AN ASTRINGENT TO ASSIST WITH CLOSING TISSUE DAMAGE. ADD FESH LEAVES TO A SACRAL STEAM OR COMPRESS, MAY ALSO BE USED IN A PERIBOTTLE TO RINSE AFTER USING THE RESTROOM
WITCH HAZEL Hamamelis Virginiana L	ASTRINGENT, ANTI-INFLAMMATORY, MILD ANTIBACTERIAL. CONTAINS CHEMICALS CALLED TANNINS. WHEN APPLIED DIRECTLY TO THE SKIN, MIGHT HELP REDUCE SWELLING, HELP REPAIR BROKEN SKIN, AND FIGHT BACTERIA. USED OFTEN IN STEAM OR COMPRESS
GUAVA LEAF Psidium guajava L	DISINFECTING ANTIMICROBIAL. USE IN A SITZ BATH OR STEAM. IS EFFECTIVE IN TREATING VAGINAL DISCHARGE. HELPFUL IN CASES OF TRICHOMONIASIS AND CANDIDIASIS. USED IN PERIBOTTLE BLEND AFTER USING THE RESTROOM OR AS A REGIMEN ONCE A DAY FOR ONE WEEK WHEN THERE IS DISCHARGE AND ODOR
AVOCADO Persea Americana	ASTRINGENT, EMOLLIENT, AND DIURETIC. IT IS USED IN INFUSIONS AND VAGINAL WASHES. ADD A HANDFUL OF FRESH LEAVES TO A VAGINAL STEAM, COMPRESS, OR BATH
EUCALYPTUS Eucalyptus Globulus	DISINFECTING, ANTIMICROBIAL, ANTISEPTIC. USED IN STEAMS, COMPRESS, AND BATHS. NOT FOR INTERNAL USE IF PREGNANT AND BREASTFEEDING.
WORMWOOD Artemisia Absinthium	AIDES IN DISINFECTING WOUNDS AND LACERATIONS AFTER CHILDBIRTH. CONTRAINDICATED FOR INGESTION DURING PREGNANCY IN THERAPEUTIC DOSES. CULINARY USE IS FINE. CONSIDERED SAFE FOR BREASTFEEDING. USE FRESH HERB IN BATH, COMPRESS OR MASSAGE OIL. TOAST WITH TOBACCO LEAVES AND MASSAGE TO WARM THE BELLY AND EASE AFTERPAINS
MUGWORT Artemisia Spp. (vulgaris, ludoviciana mexicana)	DIURETIC, DIGESTIVE, EXPECTORANT, ANTISEPTIC, DIAPHORETIC, ANTISPASMODIC, ANTI-INFLAMMATORY, ANALGESIC. USED AS A STEAM, POULTICE, INFUSION, BATH OR MASSAGE OIL IN MEXICAN TRADITIONAL MEDICINE, ESPECIALLY FOR POSTPARTUM PRACTICE. INGESTION IS CONTRAINDICATED DURING PREGNANCY AND BREASTFEEDING. USED TO REDUCE SWELLING AND EASE AFTERPAINS.

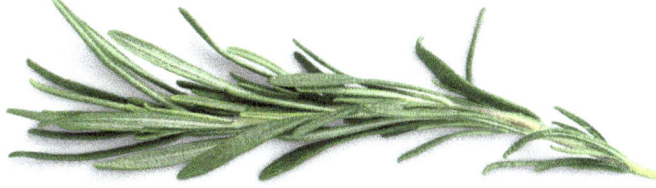

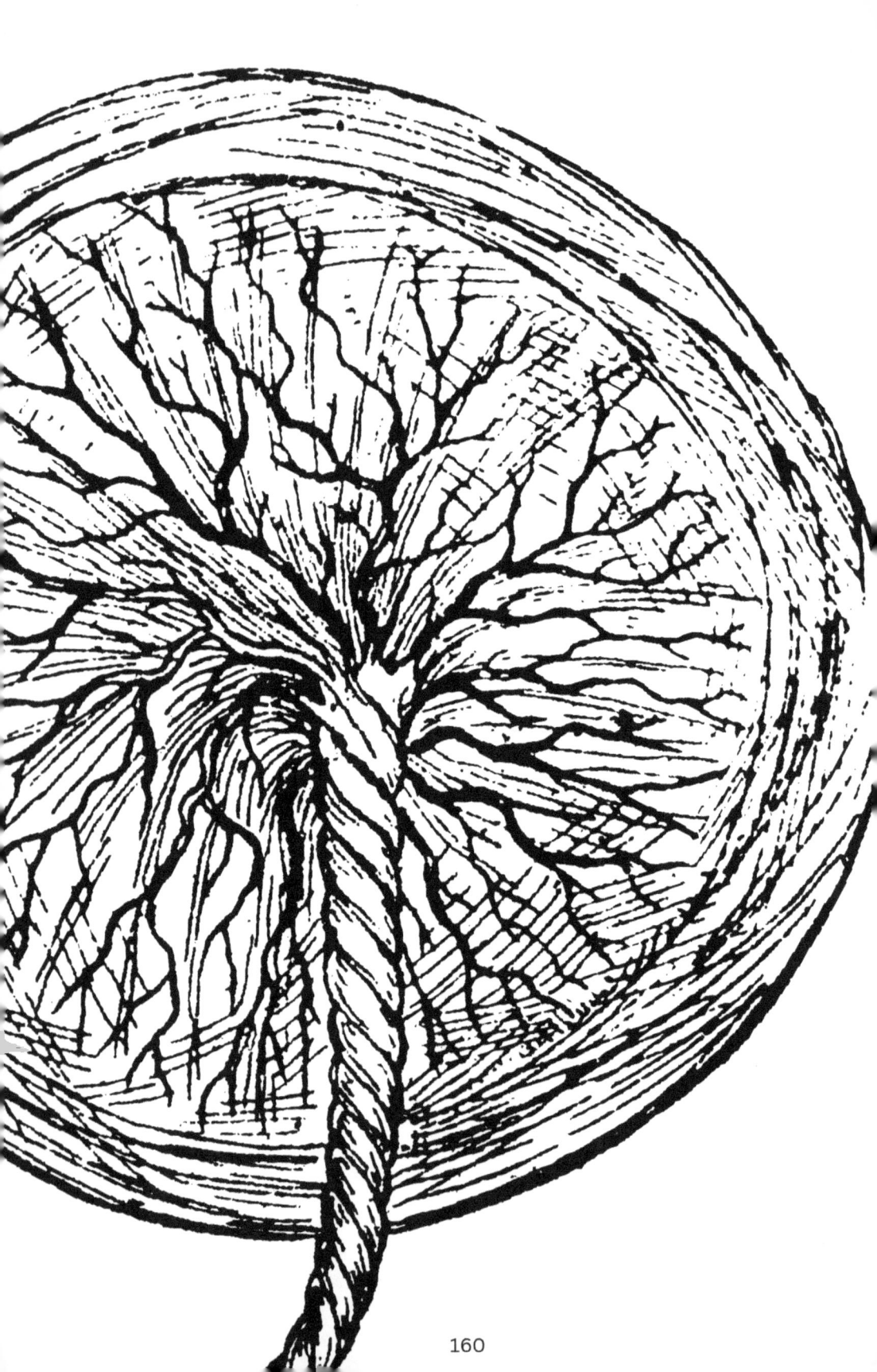

Honoring The Placenta

Honoring the placenta is a practice with profound cultural and spiritual significance, observed in various ways across the globe. Here are examples of traditional placenta rituals:

1. Japan: In Japan, the placenta, known as "*ochiai*," is traditionally buried in the garden of the family home. This burial is often accompanied by a small ceremony, and sometimes a tree or plant is planted over the spot to symbolize growth and continuity, nurturing both the child and the placenta.

2. Haiti: In Haitian culture, the placenta is buried in a sacred or designated area, often under a tree. This act is accompanied by prayers or rituals to ensure the well-being of the mother and child, with the location often chosen for its spiritual significance.

3. New Zealand: Among the Māori people of New Zealand, the placenta is buried in a special place known as "*papakainga*" or "ancestral land." This practice reflects the deep connection between the child, the family, and the land, honoring the placenta's role and reinforcing the bond with ancestors.

4. Philippines: In some Filipino communities, the placenta is buried near the family home in a designated spot. This practice is believed to ensure good fortune and health for the child. Rituals may include prayers or offerings to honor the placenta.

5. Ghana: In Ghana, the placenta is sometimes buried in the family home's compound or another traditional location. The burial is accompanied by rituals and offerings to honor the placenta and invoke blessings for the child and family.

6. Australia: Among some Aboriginal communities, the placenta is buried in a culturally significant location. This practice is part of a broader set of rituals emphasizing the connection between the child, the land, and the ancestors.

7. China: Traditional Chinese Medicine (TCM) has long utilized the placenta for medicinal purposes. The placenta may be dried, powdered, and encapsulated for ingestion, believed to balance hormones, accelerate postpartum recovery, and support overall health. It may also be buried with rituals to ensure the child's well-being.

8. United States: In the U.S., placenta encapsulation has become popular. This process involves dehydrating and encapsulating the placenta for ingestion, which is believed to offer benefits such as improved mood, enhanced energy, and faster postpartum recovery. Some practitioners also make placenta tinctures for long-term health benefits, including support during menopause.

9. Ecuador: Among Indigenous communities in Ecuador, the placenta is considered a twin companion to the child. If either the mother or child falls ill, it is important to tend to both the affected individual and the plant buried atop the placenta. This reflects the belief in the placenta's spiritual and physical connection to the family's health.

10. Navajo: The Navajo people often bury the placenta in a sacred location,

such as beneath a tree or within a ceremonial space. This ritual emphasizes the connection between the child and the earth, reinforcing the child's place within the natural and spiritual realms.

The practices of placenta encapsulation and ingestion, alongside traditional burial or ceremonial rites, highlight the continued reverence for this organ. The diverse ways in which cultures honor the placenta underscore its importance in the childbirth journey and its symbolic role in connecting life, health, and spirituality.

Ingesting the placenta is rooted in ancient traditions and has gained popularity in recent decades for its potential health benefits. Historical use of the placenta for medicinal purposes dates back to 16th-century China, where it was believed to balance hormones, accelerate recovery, and improve overall well-being. Modern studies have examined these claims, finding that encapsulated placenta contains iron and trace minerals. While its impact on postpartum mood disorders and recovery remains debated, some studies have identified various hormones in placenta capsules, suggesting potential physiological effects, though typically at low concentrations.

There are many variations for the preparation of placenta. It may be steamed with food such as lemon, jalapeño, red peppers, and chilies. Or with herbs like ginger, frankincense, myrrh, lemon grass, garlic, turmeric, and white peony root. TCM preparation includes a practitioner consultation to discern the birthing person's specific needs and create a customized herbal blend. When deciding what herbs will best compliment the properties of the placenta, always choose herbs that have similar actions and assist with the transitions experienced in postpartum.

The placenta can also be tinctured. The tincture can be used for postaprtum or saved for menopausal support. Ashwagandha , vitex, black cohosh, and motherwort are herbs used in transition tinctures.

The impact of consuming placenta can vary depending on both the quality of the placenta and the mother's overall health. Placenta ingestion is generally contraindicated if the mother tests positive for Group B Streptococcus, HIV, Hepatitis B or C, or any active infections due to the risk of transmitting these conditions. To enhance the benefits of placenta encapsulation, many practitioners include warming herbs in the process. These herbs are believed to support postpartum healing by helping to restore balance and promote overall recovery. Additionally, placenta tinctures, which are prepared by extracting the placenta's essence into a liquid form, can be stored for long-term use. These tinctures may provide ongoing support during menopause, offering potential benefits such as hormonal balance and overall well-being. Overall, the practice of honoring the placenta reflects a deep respect for its significance in the postpartum journey and its role in the well-being of both mother and child.

HERBS FOR PLACENTA ENCAPSULATION

PREPARATION OF HERBS:
WASH AND PEEL THE FRESH GINGER. SLICE IT THINLY TO MAXIMIZE THE SURFACE AREA.
COMBINE THE FRESH GINGER SLICES WITH THE DRIED HERBS IN A MIXING BOWL.

ENCAPSULATION:
USING A DEHYDRATOR, SPREAD THE GINGER AND ANY OTHER FRESH HERBS EVENLY ON THE TRAYS AND DEHYDRATE AT A LOW TEMPERATURE (95-105°F OR 35-40°C) UNTIL COMPLETELY DRY. THIS MAY TAKE SEVERAL HOURS AND IS USUALLY DONE IN TANDEM WITH THE PLACENTA).
ONCE DRIED, ADD OTHER ALREADY DRIED HERBS AND GRIND THE MIXTURE INTO A FINE POWDER USING A HERB GRINDER OR A HIGH-QUALITY BLENDER.
ENCAPSULATE THE POWDER INTO EMPTY CAPSULES.

STORAGE:
STORE THE ENCAPSULATED HERBS IN A COOL, DRY PLACE, AWAY FROM DIRECT SUNLIGHT.

USAGE:
WEEK 1: TAKE 2 CAPSULES 3 TIMES PER DAY
WEEK 2: TAKE 2 CAPSULES 2 TIMES PER DAY
WEEK 3: TAKE 1 CAPSULE 2 TIMES PER DAY
WEEK 4-6: TAKE 1 CAPSULE 1 TIME PER DAY

BOTH THE CAPSULES AND TINCTURES CAN BE USED TO SUPPORT HORMONAL BALANCE AND ALLEVIATE PERIMENOPAUSAL SYMPTOMS.
MAKING IT A SUPPORTIVE ADDITION TO POSTPARTUM CARE AND PERIMENOPAUSE MANAGEMENT.

PLACENTA BLENDS FOR POSTPARTUM

HERBS / REMEDIES:
FRESH GINGER PROMOTES CIRCULATION AND AIDS RECOVERY;
GOJI BERRIES NOURISH BLOOD AND SUPPORT LIVER AND KIDNEY HEALTH
RED DATES BOOST ENERGY AND AID POSTPARTUM RECOVERY
CINNAMON WARMS THE BODY AND SUPPORTS CIRCULATION

POWDERED POSTPARTUM BLEND
- 2 PART FRESH GINGER (SHENG JIANG, ZINGIBER OFFICINALE)
- 1 PART GOJI BERRIES (GOU QI ZI, LYCIUM BARBARUM)
- 1 PART RED DATES (JUJUBE, DA ZAO, ZIZIPHUS JUJUBA)
- ¼ PART CINNAMON TWIG (GUI ZHI, CINNAMOMUM CASSIA)

THIS TCM-INSPIRED BLEND INTEGRATES WARMING AND HARMONIZING HERBS TO SUPPORT POSTPARTUM RECOVERY AND PERIMENOPAUSAL HEALTH, ALIGNING WITH TRADITIONAL PRINCIPLES OF BALANCING THE BODY'S ENERGY AND ENHANCING OVERALL WELL-BEING.

TINCTURED POSTPARTUM BLEND
- 2 PART FRESH GINGER
- ½ PART MOTHERWORT
- ¼ PART CINNAMON
- ¼ PART ROSE PETALS

SUPPORTS POSTPARTUM RECOVERY BY EASING DISCOMFORT, PROMOTING HORMONAL BALANCE, AND SOOTHING ANXIETY. IT ENHANCES DIGESTIVE HEALTH, STABILIZES BLOOD SUGAR LEVELS, AND IMPROVES CIRCULATION WHILE ALSO PROVIDING EMOTIONAL SUPPORT AND PROMOTING SKIN HEALTH.

FRESH GINGER FOR ITS WARMING AND DIGESTIVE SUPPORT, MOTHERWORT FOR UTERINE HEALTH AND MOOD BALANCE, CINNAMON FOR IMPROVING CIRCULATION AND STABILIZING BLOOD SUGAR, AND ROSE PETALS FOR EMOTIONAL CALM

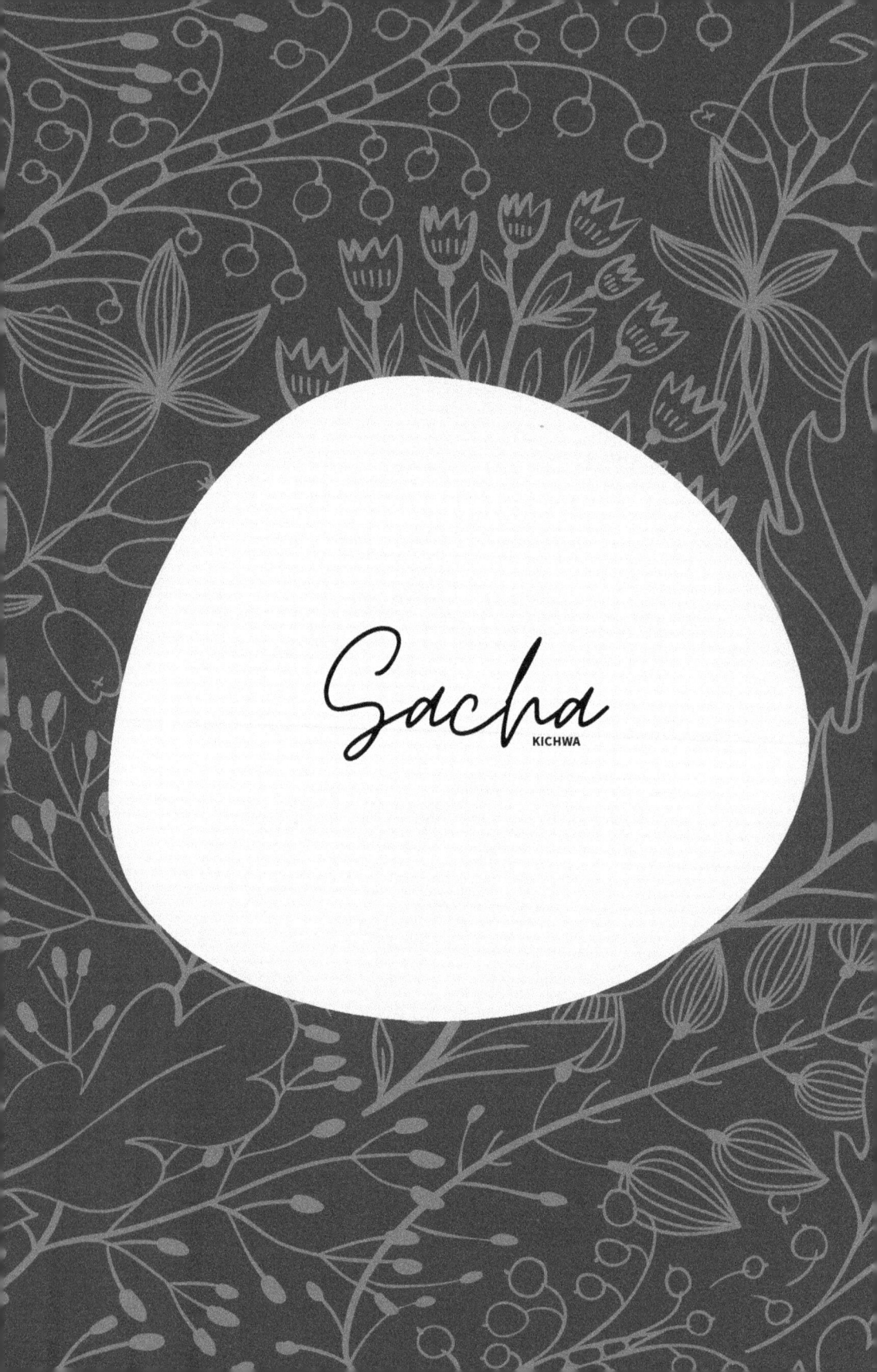

BIRTH AS A SUSTO

"Susto" is a term used in traditional Latin American and Indigenous cultures to describe a condition where a person experiences a sudden fright or shock so intense that it is believed their spirit or soul temporarily leaves the body. This concept, rooted in spiritual and cultural beliefs, often occurs after a severe stress, or a significant emotional disturbance. Those who suffer from susto may exhibit symptoms such as anxiety, depression, fatigue, loss of appetite, and a sense of disconnection or emptiness. As beautiful as it is, many still see birth as a form of "susto," where the spirit temporarily leaves the body. In this context, susto is the spirit is departure to fetch the soul of the baby, returning with it to complete the profound journey of childbirth. This belief highlights the need to intentionally call the mother's spirit back into her body after birth, ensuring her full presence and well-being as she steps into the new chapter of motherhood.

In traditional healing practices, susto is support through rituals and remedies aimed at calling the spirit back to the body and restoring balance and harmony to the individual's life. These might include cleansing rituals, prayers, herbal remedies, and other forms of spiritual healing conducted by a healer or curandero. The condition is recognized as both a physical and spiritual ailment, requiring a holistic approach to healing.

This is where post-birth ceremonies become so important. Grounding herbs, heart-opening rituals, and practices like the "Closing the Bones" ceremony play a crucial role in helping the mother reclaim her spirit and integrate the transformative experience of giving birth.

The Closing the Bones ceremony, practiced in various cultures, involves gently wrapping and massaging the mother's body to symbolically and physically seal her spirit back into her body. This ritual not only provides physical comfort but also marks the mother's emergence from the bindings as a rebirth into her new role, sealing the experience of birth and acknowledging her transition. Symbolically closing the energy field and guiding the spirit back into alignment helps prevent postpartum mood disorders that can arise when the spirit remains ungrounded, creating an opening for imbalance.

Acknowledging the heart, spirit, mind, and body of a new mother is integral to holistic healing. Supporting all aspects of her being helps to create a strong foundation for her new life chapter.

HEART OPENER HERBS

ASHWAGANDHA (WITHANIA SOMNIFERA) - IN AYURVEDA, ASHWAGANDHA IS USED TO STRENGTHEN THE HEART, REDUCE STRESS, AND ENHANCE EMOTIONAL RESILIENCE.

BAOBAB (ADANSONIA DIGITATA) - REVERED IN MANY AFRICAN CULTURES, BAOBAB IS RICH IN NUTRIENTS THAT SUPPORT OVERALL VITALITY AND IS SOMETIMES USED TO STRENGTHEN THE HEART AND SPIRIT.

CACAO (THEOBROMA CACAO) - CENTRAL TO MESOAMERICAN CULTURES, CACAO IS USED IN CEREMONIAL CONTEXTS TO OPEN THE HEART AND CONNECT WITH THE DIVINE.

DAMIANA (TURNERA DIFFUSA) - USED BY THE INDIGENOUS PEOPLES OF CENTRAL AND SOUTH AMERICA AS AN APHRODISIAC AND HEART OPENER.

HAWTHORN (CRATAEGUS SPP.) - A SACRED PLANT IN EUROPEAN TRADITIONS, ESPECIALLY CELTIC, USED TO STRENGTHEN AND PROTECT THE HEART.

HIBISCUS (HIBISCUS SABDARIFFA) - WIDELY USED ACROSS AFRICA, PARTICULARLY IN WEST AFRICA, HIBISCUS IS KNOWN FOR ITS COOLING, CALMING PROPERTIES THAT SUPPORT HEART HEALTH.

JASMINE (JASMINUM SAMBAC) - IN AYURVEDIC AND TRADITIONAL CHINESE MEDICINE, JASMINE IS USED TO UPLIFT THE HEART AND SOOTHE THE MIND, OFTEN IN THE FORM OF TEA OR OIL.

KANNA (SCELETIUM TORTUOSUM) - INDIGENOUS TO SOUTH AFRICA, KANNA HAS BEEN USED BY THE SAN AND KHOIKHOI PEOPLE FOR ITS MOOD-LIFTING AND HEART-OPENING EFFECTS.

LAVENDER (LAVANDULA SPP.) - WIDELY USED IN MEDITERRANEAN CULTURES, LAVENDER PROMOTES RELAXATION AND EMOTIONAL HEALING.

LEMON BALM (MELISSA OFFICINALIS) - A CALMING HERB USED IN EUROPEAN AND MIDDLE EASTERN TRADITIONS TO SOOTHE THE HEART AND UPLIFT THE MOOD.

LINDEN (TILIA SPP.) - A BELOVED REMEDY IN EUROPEAN FOLK MEDICINE, ESPECIALLY IN SLAVIC COUNTRIES, FOR CALMING THE NERVES AND OPENING THE HEART.

LOTUS (NELUMBO NUCIFERA) - SACRED IN MANY ASIAN CULTURES, PARTICULARLY IN INDIA AND CHINA, LOTUS IS USED TO CALM THE HEART, BALANCE EMOTIONS, AND PROMOTE SPIRITUAL CLARITY.

MOTHERWORT (LEONURUS CARDIACA) - TRADITIONALLY USED IN CHINESE AND WESTERN HERBAL MEDICINE TO CALM THE HEART AND EASE ANXIETY.

REISHI MUSHROOM (GANODERMA LUCIDUM) - KNOWN AS "LINGZHI" IN CHINA AND "MANNENTAKE" IN JAPAN, REISHI IS REVERED IN TRADITIONAL CHINESE MEDICINE AS A HEART TONIC THAT PROMOTES EMOTIONAL AND SPIRITUAL WELL-BEING.

ROSE (ROSA SPP.) - USED IN MANY CULTURES, INCLUDING PERSIAN AND WESTERN HERBALISM, FOR ITS CALMING AND HEART-OPENING PROPERTIES.

SHATAVARI (ASPARAGUS RACEMOSUS) - ANOTHER IMPORTANT HERB IN AYURVEDA, SHATAVARI IS USED TO NOURISH THE HEART, BALANCE HORMONES, AND SUPPORT EMOTIONAL HEALTH, ESPECIALLY IN WOMEN.

TULSI/HOLY BASIL (OCIMUM SANCTUM) - REVERED IN INDIAN AYURVEDA, TULSI IS BELIEVED TO OPEN THE HEART AND UPLIFT THE SPIRIT.

YARROW (ACHILLEA MILLEFOLIUM) - KNOWN IN EUROPEAN AND NATIVE AMERICAN TRADITIONS FOR ITS ABILITY TO HEAL EMOTIONAL WOUNDS AND PROTECT THE HEART.

HEART OPENER FORMULAS

THESE BLENDS ARE WARM, SOOTHING DRINKS TO NOURISH THE BODY AND OPENS YOUR HEART, MAKING IT PERFECT FOR RELAXATION AND EMOTIONAL CONNECTION.

HERB/REMEDIES: MOTHERWORT EASES ANXIETY AND SUPPORTS UTERINE HEALTH, WHILE HAWTHORN STRENGTHENS THE HEART. SHATAVARI BALANCES HORMONES, ASHWAGANDHA REDUCES STRESS, AND SKULLCAP CALMS THE NERVOUS SYSTEM, MAKING THIS BLEND IDEAL FOR POSTPARTUM HEART-OPENING SUPPORT.

TINCTURE
- 1 PART MOTHERWORT
- ½ PART HAWTHORNE
- ½ PART SHATAVARI
- ½ PART ASHWAGANDA
- ½ PART SKULLCAP

THIS HEART-OPENING BLEND FEATURES HOLY BASIL FOR ITS UPLIFTING AND CALMING EFFECTS, DAMIANA FOR ENHANCING EMOTIONAL WELL-BEING, SKULLCAP FOR EASING NERVOUS TENSION, LINDEN FOR SOOTHING THE HEART, AND ROSE FOR ITS CALMING AND SUPPORTIVE PROPERTIES.

TEA
1 PART HOLY BASIL
1 PART DAMIANA
1 PART SKULLCAP
1 PART LINDEN
¼ PART ROSE

CACAO BLEND

CACAO, RICH IN ANTIOXIDANTS, MAGNESIUM, AND IRON, SUPPORTS VITALITY, REDUCES STRESS, ENHANCES MOOD, AND IS TRADITIONALLY USED TO OPEN THE HEART AND FOSTER EMOTIONAL CONNECTION. DAMIANA, KNOWN FOR ITS CALMING AND APHRODISIAC PROPERTIES, EASES ANXIETY, UPLIFTS THE SPIRIT, AND OPENS THE HEART, WHILE COCONUT MILK NOURISHES THE BODY WITH HEALTHY FATS THAT SUSTAIN ENERGY.

INGREDIENTS:
- 2 TABLESPOONS RAW CACAO POWDER
- 1 TEASPOON DRIED DAMIANA LEAVES
- 1 CUP COCONUT MILK
- 1 TABLESPOON HONEY OR MAPLE SYRUP
- ½ TEASPOON CINNAMON
- ¼ TEASPOON VANILLA EXTRACT)
- PINCH OF CAYENNE PEPPER

STEEP DAMIANA LEAVES IN SIMMERING WATER FOR 10 MINUTES, THEN STRAIN. WARM COCONUT MILK, THEN WHISK IN CACAO, CINNAMON, VANILLA, AND CAYENNE. COMBINE WITH DAMIANA TEA, SWEETEN IF DESIRED, AND SERVE.

THIS DRINK ALSO SUPPORTS POSTPARTUM RECOVERY BY EASING DISCOMFORT, PROMOTING HORMONAL BALANCE, SOOTHING ANXIETY, AND IMPROVING CIRCULATION AND DIGESTION.

"The world begins at a kitchen table. No matter what, we must eat to live. The gifts of earth are brought and prepared, set on the table. So it has been since creation, and it will go on."

Joy Harjo (Muscogee Creek Nation, Poet and Former U.S. Poet Laureate)

chapter 9

The Role Of Food
Global First Foods
Wellness Recipes

"Food is medicine. During pregnancy and postpartum, it's not just about eating to sustain life; it's about nourishing the body and soul, honoring the life force within."

— Robyn Morissette
Indigenous midwife and herbalist

Love You Like Cooked Food

Food for many is our first memory of love, from the breast to the plate—it is a manifestation of nurturing affection. Food is more than just fuel; it is intertwined with our daily lives and often forms the core of family and community celebrations. For many, it is also tied to our emotions, offering comfort and solace. It can be a quick journey to a place in time, a person, or a land that we hold dear.

In pregnancy and postpartum care, food holds even more significance because you are "eating for two." It is a vital source of healing and connection. .During pregnancy, a woman's body undergoes immense changes, demanding increased nourishment to support both her health and the baby's development. Consuming nutrient-dense foods rich in folate, iron, calcium, and omega-3 fatty acids is crucial for fetal development and maternal well-being. Whole foods like leafy greens, lean proteins, whole grains, nuts, seeds, and fresh fruits and vegetables are prepared with reverence and gratitude, ensuring that the life-giving energy within them supports both mother and baby.

In the postpartum period, the body requires significant replenishment to recover not only from childbirth but also from pregnancy, and it needs to be fortified for the demands of nurturing a new life. Postpartum nutrition aims not just to heal but to restore and strengthen. Many cultures emphasize warm, easily digestible, and nutrient-rich foods, such as soups, stews, and broths made from nutritive fats, fresh vegetables, and infused herbs. These foods offer essential hydration, warmth, and nourishment. By replenishing depleted nutrients and restoring balance, postpartum eating helps fortify the mother, preparing her to meet the challenges of life with renewed strength and vitality.

Micronutrients in food and herbs play a vital role in enriching maternal and fetal health. Herbs like ginger and turmeric provide anti-inflammatory and digestive benefits, while nettle and red raspberry leaf supply essential vitamins and minerals. When these herbs are carefully gathered and prepared with intention, the food is enriched with both nutrients and purpose. Thus, the spirit of the food—whether in the form of a healing broth or a nourishing herbal tea—boosts physical, and emotional well-being.

Eating has always been more than just calories converting to energy, and food during pregnancy and postpartum is more than just sustenance. It is a sacred practice that supports the health and well-being of both mother and baby. Eating becomes a profound ritual of nurturing that fortifies the body, mind, and spirit, bridging the physical and spiritual realms, and nurturing the entire family during one of life's most transformative transitions.

Adding Herbs To Food

Incorporating medicinal herbs into your food can be simple and rewarding, enhancing flavor while delivering a range of health benefits. Here are easy and practical ways to include medicinal herbs in your cooking:

1. Make It A Decoction: Add Dried Roots, Berries, and Barks to Simmering Pots
Their medicinal properties are released during the long simmering process just as they would in a decoction.
Can be used in both base broths and soups or while cooking grains and beans.
Example: Dried roots like burdock and astragalus can be powerful additions to base broths and soups. Burdock root is known for its detoxifying properties, while Astragalus root supports immunity. Simply add the dried roots to your pot and let them simmer alongside other ingredients.

2. Incorporate Dried Herbs into Dishes
Adding dried herbs to dishes like beans or grains can aid in digestion and offer anti-inflammatory benefits infusing them with flavor and medicinal benefits:
Example: Add dried herbs like thyme to beans while cooking or sprinkle in herbs like cilantro or oregano when cooking grains like rice or quinoa. These herbs can aid in digestion and offer anti-inflammatory benefits.

3. Sprinkle Seaweed for Flavor and Nutrients
Seaweed is a seed vegetable and high in trace minerals and nutrients not found in other foods. Adding it to broths, beans and grains as well as sprinkling onto of food as a seasoning will offer a rich source of minerals and a unique flavor:
Example: Sprinkle seaweed flakes over soups, salads, or stir-fries for added flavor and nutrients. Seaweeds are high in iodine, which supports thyroid function, and provide a range of essential minerals.

4. Use Fresh Herbs for Gentle Detoxification
Fresh herbs can be easily incorporated into your daily meals for their detoxifying and health-promoting effects:
Example: Add fresh cilantro to salads, salsas, or smoothies. Cilantro is known for its gentle detoxifying properties, helping to remove heavy metals from the body. Fresh mint can be used in teas or added to salads and yogurt. It supports digestion and adds a refreshing flavor.

5. Enhance Microbial Health with Garlic
Garlic has strong antimicrobial properties and is helpful to combat illness at the onset of cold or flu symptoms. Combine with lemon, few slices of raw ginger and honey and mash or puree in a blender. Garlic is believed to be a galactagogue and has been used for many years as an herbal remedy to stimulate breast milk production and increase the supply of breast milk. This may be because babies like the flavor and spend more time at the breast stimulating the breast to produce more milk (more demand equals more supply) . One study found that babies nursed more often and ingested more milk when mothers took a garlic supplement before nursing.

Garlic can be used in a variety of dishes:
Raw Garlic: Mince raw garlic and add it to salad dressings or marinades to maximize its health benefits. Garlic supports immune system function and helps combat harmful microbes.
Cooked Garlic: Incorporate garlic into soups, stews, and stir-fries. While cooking may reduce some of its potency, garlic still offers substantial health benefits when used regularly.

6. Create Herb-Infused Pestos and Sauces
Medicinal herbs can be blended into pestos and sauces to boost their nutritional profile:
Example: Blend moringa leaves with garlic, nuts, olive oil, and lemon juice to create a nutrient-rich pesto. Moringa is packed with vitamins, minerals, and antioxidants, making it a powerful addition to your diet. Use herbs like basil, oregano, and thyme to make flavorful sauces and depth to your dishes while contributing medicinal properties.

7. Enhance Smoothies and Juices
Medicinal herbs can be seamlessly added to smoothies and juices for an extra health boost:
Example: Add a handful of chickweed or nettle to your smoothies. These herbs are rich in vitamins and minerals that support overall health. Infuse juices with herbs like ginger or turmeric. These herbs offer anti-inflammatory benefits and can enhance the flavor of your juice.

"In our culture, food is central to every stage of life, especially in pregnancy and postpartum. It's about more than just nutrition; it's about ritual, family, and healing."

– Aurora Garcia, Traditional Mexican Midwife

Nourishment

The first meal after childbirth holds profound significance for both physical recovery and emotional well-being. Often referred to as the "first foods" in many cultures, this meal symbolizes the beginning of a new chapter and serves multiple vital purposes. Physically, it is crucial for replenishing essential nutrients lost during labor and delivery. This meal typically includes proteins for tissue repair, iron to restore blood levels, and vitamins and minerals to support overall healing, with nutrient-dense foods like lean meats, leafy greens, and whole grains being emphasized. Given the physical demands of labor, the first meal also plays a key role in restoring energy levels, with carbohydrates and healthy fats providing a quick source of energy for the new mother. Additionally, the first meal supports lactation, with foods rich in omega-3 fatty acids, calcium, and protein—such as salmon, nuts, and dairy products—helping to ensure a healthy milk supply.

Beyond its physical benefits, the first meal after childbirth offers emotional and psychological support. Comforting and familiar foods can provide emotional reassurance, offering a sense of normalcy and easing the transition into motherhood during a time of significant change. Sharing this meal with family or close friends can be a celebratory event, marking the arrival of the new baby and acknowledging the mother's strength and resilience. This communal aspect reinforces social support and fosters a sense of connection and celebration.

The cultural significance of the first meal is also profound. Many cultures have specific traditions and rituals associated with it, often involving special ingredients believed to have healing properties or symbolic meanings. These traditions honor cultural heritage and offer spiritual and emotional support to the new mother, with the meal often holding symbolic importance as a way to welcome the mother and baby into the world with nourishment and care. This aligns with cultural beliefs about the sacred nature of food and its role in healing.

The first meal is designed to be easy to prepare and digest. Simple, well-cooked, and easily digestible foods ensure that it can be enjoyed without added stress. Hydration is also crucial, with adequate fluid intake supporting postpartum recovery and milk production. Soups, broths, or herbal teas can complement the first meal, providing additional hydration.

The first meal can play an impactful role in the postpartum experience, helping to ease the transition into motherhood and support the well-being of both mother and baby.

Global First Foods

These traditional postpartum meals reflect the rich cultural heritage of various regions and provide essential nutrients and comfort to support recovery during the postpartum period. Each dish is crafted with care to nourish the body, mind, and spirit as new mothers transition into this transformative phase.

Atole (Mexico)
Description: Atole is a traditional Mexican beverage made from masa (corn dough), water or milk, and sweetened with piloncillo (unrefined cane sugar) or sugar. It can be flavored with cinnamon, vanilla, or chocolate.
Benefits: Atole is warm and comforting, providing essential carbohydrates for energy. The corn base is easy to digest and offers gentle nourishment, making it a soothing drink during the postpartum period.

Borscht (Russia/Ukraine)
Description: Borscht is a beet soup that often includes vegetables, beef, and sometimes beans. it is typically served with a dollop of sour cream.
Benefits: Beets are rich in iron and vitamins, which help in replenishing blood and supporting recovery. The soup's warm nature is soothing and provides comfort during postpartum.

Chicken and Ginseng Soup (Korea)
Description: Known as "Samgyetang," this soup features a whole young chicken stuffed with ginseng, garlic, jujube dates, and glutinous rice, then simmered until tender.
Benefits: Ginseng is renowned for its restorative properties, supporting energy and immune function. The chicken provides protein and essential nutrients, while the broth offers warmth and helps with recovery.

Coconut Milk Rice (Southeast Asia)
Description: Rice cooked with coconut milk and sometimes infused with herbs like pandan or lemongrass.
Benefits: Coconut milk provides healthy fats and energy, while the rice is a good source of carbohydrates. The addition of herbs can offer additional nutrients and a soothing, comforting quality.

Congee (China)
Description: Congee is a warm, rice porridge often made with chicken, pork, or fish and cooked until very soft. It can be flavored with ginger, scallions, and other herbs.
Benefits: This dish is easily digestible and provides gentle nourishment. It's rich in carbohydrates for energy, and ingredients like ginger and chicken help to warm the body, support digestion, and aid in postpartum recovery.

Khichdi (India)
Description: Khichdi is a comforting dish made from a mix of rice and lentils, often cooked with turmeric, ginger, and spices.
Benefits: This dish is easy to digest and provides balanced protein and carbohydrates. Turmeric and ginger have anti-inflammatory properties that support healing and digestion.

Kitchari (Ayurvedic)
Description: Kitchari is a blend of basmati rice and mung beans, cooked with ghee and spices like cumin, coriander, and turmeric.
Benefits: Mung beans are rich in protein and fiber, while ghee aids in digestion and provides essential fats. This dish is easy on the digestive system and supports detoxification and energy levels.

Moringa Soup (West Africa)
Description: This soup is made from moringa leaves, which are often cooked with meats such as goat or chicken, along with tomatoes, onions, and spices.
Benefits: Moringa leaves are highly nutritious, offering a rich source of vitamins, minerals, and antioxidants. The soup helps replenish nutrients, boosts milk production, and provides energy.

Nettle Soup (Europe)
Description: Nettle soup is made from fresh nettle leaves, onions, garlic, and sometimes potatoes or cream.
Benefits: Nettle is a nutrient powerhouse, offering high levels of vitamins and minerals like iron, which help replenish energy and support milk production.

Pozole (Mexico)
Description: Pozole is a traditional Mexican stew made from hominy corn, meat (such as pork or chicken), and spices. It is often garnished with radishes, lime, and cilantro.
Benefits: The hominy corn in pozole is high in niacin and helps to support energy levels. The dish is also a rich source of protein and vitamins, aiding in overall recovery and providing warmth and comfort during the postpartum period.

Yao Zhuo (Haiti)
Description: Yao Zhuo is a traditional Haitian dish made with a variety of meats (often goat or beef) and vegetables like okra and eggplant, cooked slowly to create a hearty stew.
Benefits: This stew is nutrient-dense, providing protein, vitamins, and minerals necessary for postpartum recovery. The slow-cooking process extracts flavors and nutrients, making it both nourishing and comforting.

FOOD RECIPES

MEDICINAL HERBAL SACHETS

HERBS / REMEDIES: ASTRAGALUS BOOSTS IMMUNITY AND ENERGY, BURDOCK AIDS DETOXIFICATION AND SKIN HEALTH, DANG SHEN REVITALIZES AND STRENGTHENS, AND GINGER IMPROVES CIRCULATION AND DIGESTION.

- 1 TBSP DRIED ASTRAGALUS ROOT
- 1 TBSP DRIED BURDOCK ROOT
- 1 TBSP DRIED DANG SHEN
- 1 TBSP DRIED GINGER ROOT (OPTIONAL DEPENDING ON YOUR DESIRED FLAVOR)
- 1-2 EMPTY MUSLIN OR CHEESECLOTH SACHET

CAN ALSO ADD YOUR FRESH HERBS LIKE ROSEMARY AND THYME

1. FILL SACHETS: PLACE 1-2 TABLESPOONS OF THE HERB BLEND INTO EACH MUSLIN OR CHEESECLOTH SACHET.
2. SEAL SACHETS: TIE THE SACHETS SECURELY WITH STRING OR USE PRE-MADE SACHETS WITH DRAWSTRINGS. DROP INTO A SIMMERING POT.

GOLDEN MILK

- 2" FRESH TURMERIC ROOT
- 2" FRESH GINGER ROOT
- 2" CINNAMON STICK
- 1 CARDAMOM POD
- 1 STAR ANISE
- 1 WHOLE CLOVE
- 3 BLACK PEPPERCORNS
- 1 QUART ALMOND OR COCONUT MILK
- HONEY OR AGAVE (TO TASTE)

INSTRUCTIONS:
1. GRIND TURMERIC, GINGER, CINNAMON, CARDAMOM, STAR ANISE, CLOVE, AND PEPPERCORNS INTO A THICK PASTE USING A MORTAR AND PESTLE.
2. COMBINE THE PASTE WITH MILK IN A POT. BRING TO A SIMMER, THEN REDUCE HEAT AND LET SIMMER ON LOW FOR 20 MINUTES.
3. STRAIN THE MIXTURE AND SWEETEN WITH HONEY OR AGAVE TO TASTE.
4. SERVE WARM.

NOTE: RAW HONEY IS TRADITIONALLY USED FOR POSTPARTUM CARE IN INDIGENOUS MESOAMERICAN CULTURES.

HIBISCUS & CHAMOMILE PORRIDGE

HERBS / REMEDIES: CINNAMON IS WARMING, CHAMOMILE AIDS RELAXATION, AND HIBISCUS OFFERS ANTIOXIDANTS AND IRON.

- 1 CUP ANY PREFERRED PORRIDGE GRAIN (OATS OR BUCKWHEAT)
- 2 CUPS PLANT-BASED MILK OR WATER
- 1 TBSP DRIED CHAMOMILE FLOWERS
- 1 TBSP DRIED HIBISCUS PETALS
- 1 CINNAMON STICK
- 1 TBSP HONEY OR MAPLE SYRUP
- FRESH FRUIT OR NUTS FOR TOPPING

INFUSE HERBS:
1. BOIL 2 CUPS OF WATER OR MILK, CHAMOMILE, AND HIBISCUS. SIMMER FOR 5 MINUTES. STRAIN OUT HERBS.
2. COOK PORRIDGE: RETURN LIQUID TO THE POT, ADD OATS, AND COOK UNTIL TENDER (5-10 MINUTES).
3. FLAVOR AND SERVE: STIR IN HONEY OR MAPLE SYRUP. TOP WITH FRESH FRUIT OR NUTS.

CALDO SANTO SOUP

CALDO SANTO IS A TRADITIONAL PUERTO RICAN SOUP MADE WITH COCONUT MILK, ROOT VEGETABLES LIKE YAUTÍA (TARO), YUCA (CASSAVA), AND MALANGA (YAM), OFTEN FEATURING FISH OR SEAFOOD. SEASONED WITH SOFRITO (A MIX OF ONIONS, PEPPERS, GARLIC, AND CILANTRO), ANNATTO OIL, AND SPICES, THIS RICH AND CREAMY SOUP IS BOTH FLAVORFUL AND COMFORTING. PACKED WITH ESSENTIAL VITAMINS, MINERALS, AND HEALTHY FATS, IT SUPPORTS POSTPARTUM RECOVERY BY PROVIDING ENERGY THROUGH CARBOHYDRATES AND PROTEIN. THE WARM, SOOTHING QUALITIES OF CALDO SANTO MAKE IT AN IDEAL MEAL FOR NEW MOTHERS, AIDING IN STRENGTH RESTORATION AND HEALING.

TRADITIONAL. INGREDIENT: 1 LB OF WHITE FISH (SUCH AS GROUPER OR SNAPPER), CLEANED AND CUT INTO CHUNKS
VEGAN ALTERNATIVE: TOFU OR TEMPEH CHUNKS, CHICKPEAS OR HEARTS OF PALM
1 LB OF "*VERDURAS*" ROOT VEGETABLES, PEELED AND CUBED (YAUTÍA, YUCA, MALANGA, OR ANY COMBINATION)
1 HERB SACHET
1 MEDIUM ONION, CHOPPED
1 BELL PEPPER (GREEN OR YELLOW), CHOPPED
4 CLOVES OF GARLIC, MINCED
¼ CUP OF SOFRITO (A BLEND OF ONIONS, GARLIC, PEPPERS, CILANTRO, AND CULANTRO)
2 CUPS OF COCONUT MILK (FRESH OR CANNED)
¼ CUP OF ANNATTO OIL (ACHIOTE OIL) OR OLIVE OIL
4 CUPS OF FISH OR CHICKEN BROTH (OR VEGAN BOULLION)
1 TEASPOON OF GROUND CUMIN
1 TEASPOON OF OREGANO
SALT AND PEPPER TO TASTE
1 BUNCH OF CILANTRO, CHOPPED (FOR GARNISH)
1 LIME, CUT INTO WEDGES (FOR SERVING)

INSTRUCTIONS:

IN A LARGE POT, BRING WATER TO A BOIL AND ADD THE PEELED AND CUBED ROOT VEGETABLES (YAUTÍA, YUCA, MALANGA). COOK UNTIL TENDER, ABOUT 15-20 MINUTES. DRAIN AND SET ASIDE.
IN THE SAME POT, HEAT THE ANNATTO OIL OVER MEDIUM HEAT. ADD THE CHOPPED ONION, GREEN BELL PEPPER, GARLIC, AND SOFRITO. SAUTÉ UNTIL THE VEGETABLES ARE SOFT AND FRAGRANT, ABOUT 5 MINUTES.

POUR IN THE COCONUT MILK AND FISH OR CHICKEN BROTH. ADD SACHET. STIR TO COMBINE. BRING TO A GENTLE SIMMER. THEN ADD THE GROUND CUMIN, OREGANO, SALT, AND PEPPER. STIR TO MIX THE SPICES EVENLY.

GENTLY ADD THE CHUNKS OF FISH (OR ALTERNATIVE) TO THE POT. SIMMER FOR ABOUT 10 MINUTES, OR UNTIL COOKED THROUGH AND FLAKES EASILY. ADD THE COOKED ROOT VEGETABLES BACK INTO THE POT. SIMMER FOR ANOTHER 5 MINUTES TO ALLOW THE FLAVORS TO MELD TOGETHER.

ADJUST THE SEASONING WITH MORE SALT AND PEPPER IF NEEDED. REMOVE THE POT FROM HEAT. LADLE THE SOUP INTO BOWLS, GARNISH WITH CHOPPED CILANTRO, AND SERVE WITH LIME WEDGES ON THE SIDE. THE LIME JUICE CAN BE SQUEEZED OVER THE SOUP FOR ADDED BRIGHTNESS.

VARIATIONS: YOU CAN ALSO ADD OTHER SEAFOOD LIKE SHRIMP OR CRAB FOR A RICHER FLAVOR.
THICKER SOUP: FOR A THICKER CONSISTENCY, MASH SOME OF THE ROOT VEGETABLES BEFORE ADDING THEM BACK TO THE POT.

POSTPARTUM BENEFITS:
1. TISSUE HEALING AND ENERGY RESTORATION
2. DIGESTIVE SUPPORT
3. HYDRATION AND MILK PRODUCTION
4. IMMUNE AND HORMONAL SUPPORT
5. EMOTIONAL AND PHYSICAL COMFORT

THANK YOU

I extend my deepest gratitude to my family for their patience and sacrifice while I immersed myself in this work. A heartfelt thanks to my incredible assistant for her support in making this project a reality. An endless thank you to my mother for being part of this and every project your hands have ever touched. You have continuously lifted me higher, allowing me to see further, and for that, I am forever grateful. Lastly, I honor my grandmothers and my ancestors for their wisdom and nourishing guidance.

This book was born from my own need as I entered the phase of motherhood, and I hope it serves as a valuable resource for others on a similar journey.

I've included additional resources—some that helped me and some that I created—for your exploration and enjoyment. Thank you for supporting this book and for joining me on this path.

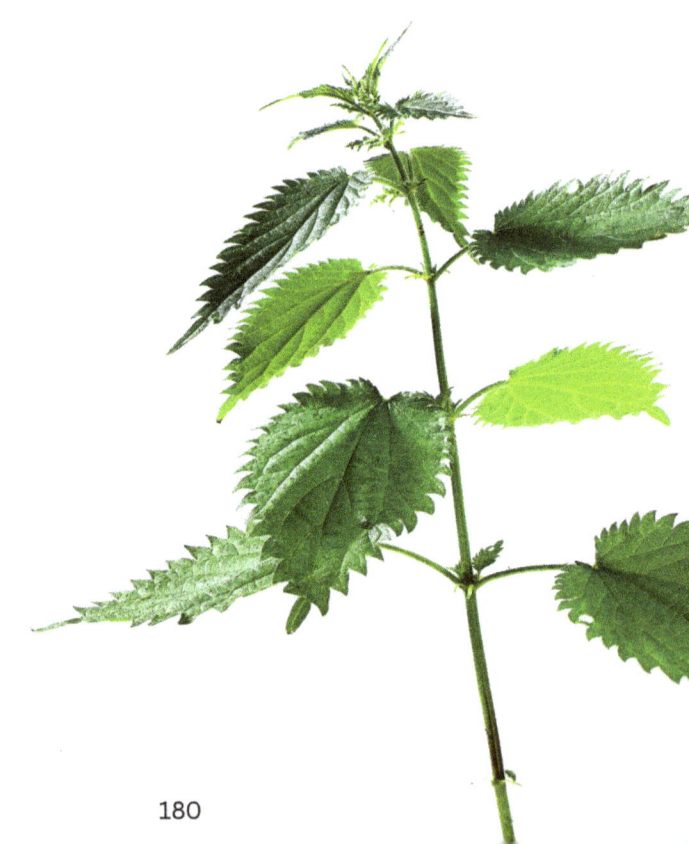

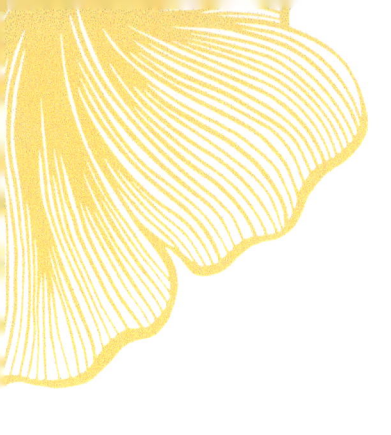

chapter 10

Herbal Safety Guide
Index and Resources

Pregnancy Safety Resource

PRE=PRECONCEPTION | PREG=PREGNANCY | BF=BREASTFEEDING

HERB	LATIN NAME	PRE	PREG	BF	ALTERNATIVE	ADDITIONAL NOTES
ACHIOTE	Bixa orellana	Y	Y	Use in culinary amount	Saffron, Turmeric, or Paprika color. Carrot (Daucus carota) for vitamin A.	ETHNOBOTANY: Achiote seeds are used in Central and South American cultures as both a spice and for medicinal purposes. PRECONCEPTION & PREGNANCY: Rich in antioxidants, supports overall health. BREASTFEEDING: Safe in culinary amounts, supports overall health. Used as natural food coloring and in traditional medicine.
ANGELICA	Angelica archangelica	Caution	N	Y	Ginger, Chamomile	PRECONCEPTION: Use with caution because it is an emmenagogue. PREGNANCY: Avoid during pregnancy due to its emmenagogue properties and because it potentially raises blood sugar.
ANISE	Pimpinella anisum	Y	Caution	Y	None	PRECONCEPTION & PREGNANCY: At therapeutic doses, anise is recognized as an emmenagogue.
ARNICA	Arnica montana	N	N	N	None	PRECONCEPTION AND PREGNANCY: Avoid arnica in therapeutic doses. EXCEPTION: Homeopathic arnica is highly diluted, which is believed to make it safer for external use.
ARTICHOKE	Cynara scolymus	Y	Y	Y	None	ETHNOBOTANY: Used in Mediterranean and European medicine for liver and digestion support. PRECONCEPTION: Supports liver detox for hormonal balance. Avoid high doses. PREGNANCY: Safe in food amounts, helps with nausea. Avoid therapeutic doses. LACTATION: Safe in food amounts, avoid concentrated extracts.
ASHWAGANDA	Withania somnifera	Y	N	Y	Ginseng, Eleuthero	ABORTIFACIENT HISTOY: Traditionally used as an abortifacient in some cultures. MALE FERTILITY: Effective in enhancing fertility and sexual performance, especially under stress.

Pregnancy Safety Resource

HERB	LATIN NAME	PRE	PREG	BF	ALTERNATIVE	ADDITIONAL NOTES
ASTRAGALUS	Astragalus membranaceous	Y	Y	Y	None	MALE FERTILITY: Traditionally used to increase the quantity & motility of sperm.
BANANA FLOWER	Musa spp.	Y	Y	Y	None	PRECONCEPTION: Supports reproductive health and hormone balance. PREGNANCY: High in fiber and nutrients, aids digestion. LACTATION: Traditionally boosts milk production. A staple in Southeast Asian and tropical diets, especially for women, often used in salads and soups.
BAOBAB	Adansonia digitata	Y	Y	Y	Acerola (Malpighia emarginata) for a high vitamin C content.	ETHNOBOTANY: Revered as the "tree of life" in African cultures. PRECONCEPTION: Provides antioxidants and supports fertility. PREGNANCY: Rich in vitamin C, enhances immune function and skin health. LACTATION: Supports overall health and replenishes vitamins. Baobab fruit pulp is highly nutritious but should be consumed in moderation.
BASIL	Ocimum basilicum	Y	Use in culinary amount	Caution	FOR DIGESTIVE SUPPORT: Thyme (Thymus vulgaris)	ETHNOBOTANY: Revered for its culinary and medicinal uses, especially in India and Southeast Asia. PREGNANCY: High doses of basil may cause miscarriage; safe in culinary amount or tea. Avoid essential oil and tincture contain carcinogenic safrole. LACTATION: Excessive basil intake may harm the nursing child; essential oil and tincture contain carcinogenic safrole.
BEARBERRY	Arctostaphylos uva-ursi	Y	N	Caution	UTI TONER: Dandelion Leaf UTI PREVENTION: Cranberry KIDNEY & BLADDER STONES: Cornsilk	PREGNANCY: This herb may stimulate contractions. LACTATION: Prolonged use during nursing may affect an infant's liver development due to its potential inhibition of B-lymphocyte cell maturation.

PRE=PRECONCEPTION
PREG=PREGNANCY
BF=BREASTFEEDING

Pregnancy Safety Resource

PRE=PRECONCEPTION   PREG=PREGNANCY   BF=BREASTFEEDING

HERB	LATIN NAME	PRE	PREG	BF	ALTERNATIVE	ADDITIONAL NOTES
BITTER MELON	*Momordica charantia*	Caution	N	Y	Jerusalem artichoke; FOR BLOOD SUGAR SUPPORT: Fenugreek (*Trigonella foenum-graecum*)	ETHNOBOTANY: Widely used in tropical Asia and Africa for its medicinal properties, particularly for managing diabetes. PRECONCEPTION: Use with caution; bitter melon is an emmenagogue. PREGNANCY: Bitter melon fruit is an emmenagogue and abortifacient.
BITTER ORANGE	*Citrus aurantium spp.*	Y	Y	Y	None	ETHNOBOTANY: Traditionally used in Chinese and Ayurvedic medicine for digestive issues and as a stimulant. PRECONCEPTION: Contains synephrine, a stimulant that may raise blood pressure and affect fertility. PREGNANCY: Avoid high doses due to its potential to increase blood pressure and uterine contractions. LACTATION: Avoid use, as stimulants may pass into breast milk and affect the infant's nervous system.
BLACK COHOSH	*Cimicifuga racemosa*	Caution	N	Caution	ANTISPASMODIC: Skullcap, Chamomile PAIN/INFLAMMATION: Rosemary HORMONE: Chaste Tree	PRECONCEPTION: Use with caution; the herb is an emmenagogue. PREGNANCY: Safe during the last weeks to prepare the uterus for contractions but unsafe at other times. LACTATION: May irritate newborns and has potential toxicity in large doses.
BLACKBERRY	*Rubus fruticosus*	Y	Y	Y	None	ETHNOBOTANY: Traditionally used in European and Native American medicine for digestive and respiratory health. PRECONCEPTION: Rich in antioxidants; supports overall reproductive health. PREGNANCY: Safe in food amounts, known to soothe digestion and ease diarrhea. LACTATION: Safe in food amounts; supports postpartum recovery due to its high nutrient content.

HERB	LATIN NAME	PRE	PREG	BF	ALTERNATIVE	ADDITIONAL NOTES
BLACKHAW VIBURNUM	Viburnum prunifolium	Y	Y	Y	None	ETHNOBOTANY: Used traditionally by Native Americans and early settlers for uterine health and as a remedy for menstrual cramps. PRECONCEPTION: Known for its antispasmodic properties; supports uterine health. PREGNANCY: Often used to prevent miscarriage and preterm labor by calming uterine contractions. LACTATION: Considered safe in moderate amounts; no known adverse effects.
BLACK WALNUT HULL	Juglans nigra	Y	Y	Y	None	ETHNOBOTANY: Traditionally used for its antiparasitic, antifungal, and antiviral properties. PRECONCEPTION: Can be a uterine stimulant and should be avoided in therapeutic doses. PREGNANCY: High tannin content can be problematic; avoid in large amounts due to its potential toxicity. LACTATION: Not recommended as it may pass harmful compounds through breast milk.
BLADDERWRACK	Fucus vesiculosus	Y	Caution	N	Sea Salt HYPO-THYROIDISM: Eleuthero CALCIUM: Red Raspberry	PREGNANCY: Excessive seaweed consumption can cause infantile goiter. Limit therapeutic doses to no more than 0.5 grams daily. LACTATION: High iodine content in seaweed may interfere with the nursing infant's thyroid function
BLESSED THISTLE	Cnicus benedictus	Y	Caution	Y	Fennel, Bitter Orange	PREGNANCY: This herb can act as an emmenagogue by irritating the digestive tract. Many thistles have been traditionally used as abortifacients.
BLUE COHOSH	Caulophyllum thalictroides	Caution	N	Y	None	PRECONCEPTION: Blue Cohosh is an emmenagogue. PREGNANCY: It is a strong uterine stimulant and can act as an abortifacient, except during the last week of pregnancy.

Pregnancy Safety Resource

PRE=PRECONCEPTION
PREG=PREGNANCY
BF=BREASTFEEDING

Pregnancy Safety Resource

BF=BREASTFEEDING
PREG=PREGNANCY
PRE=PRECONCEPTION

HERB	LATIN NAME	PRE	PREG	BF	ALTERNATIVE	ADDITIONAL NOTES
BLUE VERVAIN	*Verbana hastate*	Y	N	Y	Goldenrod, cornsilk	PREGNANCY: Can cause uterine contractions
BUCHU	*Barosma betulina*	Y	Caution	Y	Dandelion, Cranberry (*Vaccinium macrocarpon*) for urinary health.	PREGNANCY: Using diuretics to treat edema in pregnancy is theoretically problematic due to the potential reduction in plasma volume, which may decrease placental perfusion. However, studies so far have not confirmed this effect.
BURDOCK	*Arctium lappa*	Y	Y	Y	None	ETHNOBOTANY: Used traditionally in both Eastern and Western herbalism for skin health, detoxification, and as a blood purifier. PRECONCEPTION: Supports liver function and detoxification, beneficial for preconception care. PREGNANCY: Considered safe in food amounts, but avoid high doses due to its possible diuretic effects, which could lead to dehydration. LACTATION: Safe in moderate amounts, but excessive use may reduce milk supply.
BUTTERBUR	*Petasites hybridus*	Caution	N	Caution	Elecampane, Wild Cherry Bark, Cramp Bark	PRECONCEPTION: Acts as an emmenagogue. PREGNANCY: Believed to be an emmenagogue and a fetal toxin due to pyrrolizidine alkaloids.
CACAO	*Theobroma cacao*	Caution	Caution	Caution	None	PRECONCEPTION: Cocoa is safe but should be limited due to its caffeine content, similar to coffee. PREGNANCY: Monitor theobromine and caffeine intake, as high levels can increase the risk of anemia, miscarriage, and birth defects. LACTATION: Theobromine is milder, but caffeine may reduce iron levels in breast milk.
CALENDULA	*Calendula officinalis*	Y	Caution	Y	None	PREGNANCY: This herb should be used sparingly in early pregnancy, as it can have emmenagogue and abortifacient qualities during the first trimester.

Pregnancy Safety Resource

HERB	LATIN NAME	PRE	PREG	BF	ALTERNATIVE	ADDITIONAL NOTES
CALIFORNIA POPPY	*Escholtzia californica*	Y	Caution	Y	Skullcap, Valerian	PREGNANCY: This herb may stimulate the uterus due to the presence of the alkaloid cryptopine.
CAMPHOR TREE	*Cinnamomum camphora*	Caution	N	N	None	PRECONCEPTION: Essential oil acts as an emmenagogue. PREGNANCY: Camphor oil contains safrole, which is toxic to a developing fetus; it is also an emmenagogue and uterine stimulant. LACTATION: Avoid using camphor essential oil on your chest or your nursing infant's skin, as inhalation and absorption in small doses can lead to central nervous system overstimulation and seizures.
CASCARA SEGRADA	*Rhamnus purshiana*	N	N	Caution	Dandelion Root, Yellow Dock Root	PRECONCEPTION & PREGNANCY: Cascara sagrada contains genotoxins that may be mutagenic. LACTATION: Anthraquinones in cascara sagrada can transfer to breast milk, potentially causing a laxative effect in infants and exposing them to genotoxins like emodin and aloe-emodin.
CASTOR BEAN	*Ricinus communis*	Caution	N	Y	Dandelion Root, Yellow Dock Root	EXTERNAL USE: Safe for all conditions. PRECONCEPTION: Castor is an emmenagogue. PREGNANCY: The oil of the bean is sometimes used to induce labor but can cause intense intestinal cramping if taken internally and has mixed results. It should never be used internally during pregnancy due to its potential as an emmenagogue and abortifacient.
CATNIP	*Nepeta cataria*	Caution	Caution	Y	Rose, Skullcap	PRECONCEPTION: Known emmenagogue. PREGNANCY: Known emmenagogue and abortifacient; use only in small amounts and/or in tea.

PRE=PRECONCEPTION
PREG=PREGNANCY
BF=BREASTFEEDING

Pregnancy Safety Resource

PRE=PRECONCEPTION
PREG=PREGNANCY
BF=BREASTFEEDING

HERB	LATIN NAME	PRE	PREG	BF	ALTERNATIVE	ADDITIONAL NOTES
CAYENNE	*Capsicum annuum*	Y	Y	Y	None	ETHNOBOTANY: Traditionally used in various cultures for digestion, circulation, and as a stimulant to increase warmth and circulation. PRECONCEPTION: Stimulates circulation, which can be beneficial for reproductive health. PREGNANCY: Safe in culinary amounts, but excessive use may cause heartburn or digestive discomfort. LACTATION: Safe in food amounts, though excessive consumption could alter the flavor of breast milk and potentially cause discomfort in the nursing infant.
CHAMOMILE	*Matricaria recutita*	Y	Y	Y	None	PRECONCEPTION, PREGNANCY, & LACTATION: Watch for any tendencies toward ragweed allergies. While the basis for this concern is uncertain, if either the mother or baby experiences wheezing, redness, or itchy eyes after drinking a cup of tea, consider finding an alternative option. PREGNANCY: Chamomile is a smooth muscle relaxant, some herbalists caution its use in high doses during pregnancy.
CHAPPARAL	*Larrea tridentata*	N	N	N	ANTI-INFLAMMATORY, ANTIFUNGAL: Calendula URINARY ANTISEPTIC: Bearberry RESPIRATORY ANTISEPTIC: Thyme TOXIC CLEARING: Red Clover, Dandelion Root	EXTERNAL USE: Safe for external use. PRECONCEPTION & PREGNANCY: The herb is banned in the U.S. for internal use due to concerns about hepatotoxicity. LACTATION: Internal use may have a more significant negative effect on the nursing mother than on her child, potentially inhibiting RNA, protein, and lipid synthesis in the mammary gland following prolactin stimulation.
CHASTE TREE	*Vitex agnus-castus*	Y	Caution	Y	None	PREGNANCY: This herb may act as an emmenagogue; however, if there is a progesterone deficiency, it is often used to help prevent miscarriage in early pregnancy.

HERB	LATIN NAME	PRE	PREG	BF	ALTERNATIVE	ADDITIONAL NOTES
CHICKWEED	*Stellaria media*	Y	Y	Y	None	ETHNOBOTANY: Used in traditional medicine for its cooling, anti-inflammatory, and skin-soothing properties. Often applied topically for skin irritations and rashes. PRECONCEPTION: Nourishing and supportive to the body, known for its mild and nutritive properties. PREGNANCY: Generally considered safe when used as a food or mild tea, but avoid high doses as its effects during pregnancy are not well-studied. LACTATION: Safe in moderate amounts and can support overall nourishment, though excessive consumption should be avoided.
CHICORY	*Cichorium intybus*	Y	Caution	Y	None	PREGNANCY: Generally safe when used in typical food and beverage amounts; avoid excessive use.
CHINESE RED DATES	*Ziziphus jujuba*	Y	Y	Y	None	PRECONCEPTION: Nourishes blood and supports fertility. PREGNANCY: Provides essential nutrients and supports blood health. LACTATION: Can enhance milk production.
CINNAMON	*Cinnamomum zeylanicum*	Y	Y	Y	None	NOT RECOMMENDED: Not safe for use as an essential oil or alcohol extract. PRECONCEPTION & PREGNANCY: Essential oil and alcohol extract contain safrole, a known carcinogen; they are also emmenagogues and abortifacients. LACTATION: Essential oil and alcohol extract contain safrole, which is a known carcinogen.
CLOVE	*Syzygium aromaticum*	Y	Use in culinary amount	Use in culinary amounts	Cinnamon (Cinnamomum verum) for similar uses.	CAUTION: Use in moderation; high doses can be toxic. ETHNOBOTANICAL: Clove is a key spice in many tropical cuisines and has a long history in traditional medicine. PRECONCEPTION: Antimicrobial properties support reproductive health. PREGNANCY: Can be used in moderation for its antiseptic and analgesic properties. LACTATION: Safe in small amounts to support digestion.

Pregnancy Safety Resource

PRE=PRECONCEPTION
PREG=PREGNANCY
BF=BREASTFEEDING

Pregnancy Safety Resource

PRE=PRECONCEPTION PREG=PREGNANCY BF=BREASTFEEDING

HERB	LATIN NAME	PRE	PREG	BF	ALTERNATIVE	ADDITIONAL NOTES
COCONUT	*Cocos Nucifera*	Y	Y	Y	Olive oil (Olea europaea) for essential fatty acids.	ETHNOBOTANICAL: Widely used in tropical regions for food, medicine, and spiritual practices. PRECONCEPTION: Hydrates and provides essential fatty acids. PREGNANCY: Coconut water is commonly used for hydration and replenishing electrolytes; it can be consumed regularly during pregnancy. LACTATION: Coconut oil supports skin health and enhances milk production.
COFFEE	*Coffea arabica*	Caution	Caution	Caution	Non-caffeinated beverages	PRECONCEPTION: Extremely drying to cervical fluids; may burden the endocrine system and cause hormonal imbalances. PREGNANCY: Can cause anemia in mother and fetus; doses of 200 mg or more daily may increase miscarriage and birth defect risks. It crosses the placenta, potentially leading to low birth weight and preterm delivery. LACTATION: Appears in breast milk at half the maternal plasma level; can reduce iron supply and block nutrient absorption in young children.
COLTSFOOT	*Tussilago farfara*	Caution	N	Caution	Mullein	PRECONCEPTION: Coltsfoot may act as an abortifacient. PREGNANCY: Contains pyrrolizidine alkaloids, which can cause liver toxicity and may also act as an abortifacient. LACTATION: Potentially toxic glycosides may pose a risk to a nursing infant's liver. It's best to avoid prolonged use (beyond four to six weeks annually) and to avoid it altogether if there is a known liver issue.

HERB	LATIN NAME	PRE	PREG	BF	ALTERNATIVE	ADDITIONAL NOTES
COMFREY	*Symphytum officinale*	Caution	Caution	Caution	Marshmallow	PRECONCEPTION: Not recommended for internal use due to pyrrolizidine alkaloids. PREGNANCY: Potentially toxic alkaloids may pose a risk to the developing fetus's liver. Prolonged use (beyond four to six weeks annually) should be avoided, particularly in individuals with known liver issues. LACTATION: Toxic alkaloids may threaten the nursing baby's liver. Prolonged use should be avoided, and it's best to refrain from use altogether if there is a known liver issue.
CORNSILK	*Zea mays*	Y	Y	Y	None	ETHNOBOTANY: Traditionally used in various cultures for its diuretic properties and to support urinary tract health. PRECONCEPTION: Often regarded as safe and may help with kidney and bladder health. PREGNANCY: Generally considered safe in moderate amounts, can support urinary health; however, excessive use should be avoided due to potential diuretic effects. LACTATION: Believed to promote lactation and may help with fluid retention; safe in moderate doses.
CRAMP BARK	*Viburnum opulus*	Y	Y	Y	None	ETHNOBOTANY: Traditionally used by Native American tribes for its muscle-relaxant properties and to relieve menstrual cramps. PRECONCEPTION: Often used to help ease menstrual discomfort and promote uterine health. PREGNANCY: Generally considered safe in moderation, may help alleviate cramping and discomfort; however, consult a healthcare provider before use. LACTATION: Considered safe and may help with uterine tonicity and muscle relaxation during breastfeeding.
CRANBERRY	*Vaccinium vitis-idaea*	Y	Y	Y	None	ETHNOBOTANY: Used by Native Americans for urinary tract health. PRECONCEPTION: Rich in antioxidants; supports reproductive health. PREGNANCY: Safe in moderation; supports urinary health but avoid excess. LACTATION: Safe to consume; may prevent urinary infections.

Pregnancy Safety Resource

PRE=PRECONCEPTION
PREG=PREGNANCY
BF=BREASTFEEDING

Pregnancy Safety Resource

PRE=PRECONCEPTION
PREG=PREGNANCY
BF=BREASTFEEDING

HERB	LATIN NAME	PRE	PREG	BF	ALTERNATIVE	ADDITIONAL NOTES
CUCUMBER	*Cucumis sativa*	Y	Y	Y	None	ETHNOBOTANY: Traditionally consumed for hydration and cooling properties in various cultures. PRECONCEPTION: Hydrating and nutrient-rich, may support overall reproductive health. PREGNANCY: Safe to consume; provides hydration and essential nutrients, but limit excessive intake due to potential digestive discomfort. LACTATION: Safe and hydrating; may help with milk supply due to high water content.
DAMIANA	*Turnera aphrodisiaca*	Y	Y	Y	None	MALE FERTILITY: Damiana is most effective as an aphrodisiac in men when a lack of interest is linked to anxiety and depression.
DANDELION	*Taraxacum officinale*	Y	Y	Y	None	ETHNOBOTANY: Used in traditional herbal medicine for digestive support, liver health, and as a diuretic. PRECONCEPTION: Nutrient-rich; may support reproductive health and detoxification. PREGNANCY: Generally safe; supports digestion and may help alleviate water retention. Use in moderation. LACTATION: Safe; may enhance milk production and provide vital nutrients to the mother and baby.
DEVIL'S CLAW	*Harpagophytum procumbens*	Y	N	N	Turmeric (*Curcuma longa*) for anti-inflammatory benefits.	PRECONCEPTION: Supports joint health and reduces inflammation. PREGNANCY: Generally avoided due to strong effects. LACTATION: Not recommended due to insufficient safety data. ETHNOBOTANY: Native to Southern Africa, traditionally used for pain and inflammation.
DONG QUAI	*Angelica sinensis*	Y	N	Caution	None	PREGNANCY: Dong quai may encourage bleeding and acts as a menstrual and uterine stimulant. LACTATION: Avoid using the herb until postpartum bleeding has ceased, and refrain from using it during each menstrual cycle while bleeding.

HERB	LATIN NAME	PRE	PREG	BF	ALTERNATIVE	ADDITIONAL NOTES
DULSE	Rhodymenia palmetto	Y	Caution	Caution	Sea Salt HYPOTHYROIDISM: Eleuthero CALCIUM: Red Raspberry, Oatstraw	PREGNANCY: Excessive seaweed consumption can lead to infantile goiter; therapeutic doses should be limited to 0.25 grams daily. LACTATION: High doses or prolonged use may overstimulate the thyroid, and the high iodine content could pose a potential risk to a nursing infant.
ECHINACEA	Echinacea spp.	Y	Y	Y	None	ETHNOBOTANY: Traditionally used by Native American tribes for immune support and to treat infections. PRECONCEPTION: Generally considered safe; may support immune health, but caution is advised in high doses. PREGNANCY: Use with caution; limited research on safety. Consult a healthcare provider before use. LACTATION: Generally considered safe; may help support the immune system of nursing mothers and infants.
ELDER	Sambucus nigra	Y	Y	Y	None	ETHNOBOTANY: Traditionally used in European and Native American herbal medicine for its antiviral properties and to treat respiratory ailments. PRECONCEPTION: Generally safe; may support overall health, but consult with a healthcare provider for personalized advice. PREGNANCY: Use with caution; limited research on safety. Consult a healthcare provider before use, particularly in medicinal doses. LACTATION: Generally considered safe; may help support immune function and alleviate cold symptoms.
ELECAMPANE	Inula helenium	Y	Y	Y	EXTERNAL: Calendula, Thyme, Goldenseal INTERNAL: None	AVOID EXTERNAL USE DURING PRECONCEPTION, PREGNANCY, AND LACTATION: Exercise caution with external application, as it may cause contact dermatitis due to allergic hypersensitivity.

Pregnancy Safety Resource

PRE=PRECONCEPTION
PREG=PREGNANCY
BF=BREASTFEEDING

Pregnancy Safety Resource

PRE=PRECONCEPTION | PREG=PREGNANCY | BF=BREASTFEEDING

HERB	LATIN NAME	PRE	PREG	BF	ALTERNATIVE	ADDITIONAL NOTES
ELDER	*Sambucus nigra*	Y	Y	Y	None	ETHNOBOTANY: Traditionally used in European and Native American herbal medicine for its antiviral properties and to treat respiratory ailments. PRECONCEPTION: Generally safe; may support overall health, but consult with a healthcare provider for personalized advice. PREGNANCY: Use with caution; limited research on safety. Consult a healthcare provider before use, particularly in medicinal doses. LACTATION: Generally considered safe; may help support immune function and alleviate cold symptoms.
ELECAMPANE	*Inula helenium*	Y	Y	Y	EXTERNAL: Calendula, Thyme, Goldenseal INTERNAL: None	AVOID EXTERNAL USE DURING PRECONCEPTION, PREGNANCY, AND LACTATION: Exercise caution with external application, as it may cause contact dermatitis due to allergic hypersensitivity.
ELEUTHERO	*Eleutherococcus senticosus*	Y	Y	Y	None	ETHNOBOTANY: Traditionally used in Russian and Asian herbal medicine as an adaptogen to enhance physical and mental performance and support the immune system. PRECONCEPTION: May help improve stamina and reduce stress, but consult with a healthcare provider before use. PREGNANCY: Use with caution; limited research on safety during pregnancy. Consult a healthcare provider for guidance. LACTATION: Generally considered safe, but it's best to consult a healthcare provider before use, especially at therapeutic doses.
EUCALYPTUS	*Eucalyptus spp.*	Y	Y	Y	ESSENTIAL OIL: Rosemary, Thyme	USE OF ESSENTIAL OIL DURING LACTATION: Essential oil can be potentially toxic to infants through skin contact, inhalation, or ingestion, as it may stress the kidneys or impair respiratory function.
FALSE UNICORN ROOT	*Chamaelirium luteum*	Y	N	Y	None	PREGNANCY: This herb is a powerful uterine tonic that may stimulate the uterus, potentially leading to contractions if not administered by an experienced professional.

Pregnancy Safety Resource

HERB	LATIN NAME	PRE	PREG	BF	ALTERNATIVE	ADDITIONAL NOTES
FENNEL	Foeniculum vulgare	Caution	Caution	Y	Use the fruit (seed) instead of the essential oil.	USE OF FRUIT (SEED) DURING PRECONCEPTION & PREGNANCY: Generally safe as a seasoning or in tea, but in therapeutic doses, the fruit can act as an emmenagogue. ESSENTIAL OIL USE DURING PRECONCEPTION & PREGNANCY: Fennel essential oil is an emmenagogue and should be avoided. ESSENTIAL OIL USE DURING LACTATION: Absorption through the skin or inhalation of fennel essential oil may be toxic to the nursing infant
FENUGREEK	Trigonella foenum-graecum	Caution	N	Y	Bitter Orange, Dill	PRECONCEPTION: Recognized as an emmenagogue. PREGNANCY: Functions as an emmenagogue, abortifacient, and uterine stimulant.
FEVERFEW	Tanacetum parthenium	Caution	Caution	Y	Skullcap, Valerian	PRECONCEPTION: Emmenagogue. PREGNANCY: Emmenagogue; avoid therapeutic doses in early pregnancy.
FLAX	Linum usitatissimum	N	N	Y	None	PRECONCEPTION: Emmenagogue. PREGNANCY: Avoid using flax during the first trimester due to its emmenagogue properties.
FORSYTHIA	Forsythia suspense	Caution	N	Y	Elder, Shiitake	PRECONCEPTION: Emmenagogue PREGNANCY: Emmenagogue and believed to be uterine stimulant
GARLIC	Allium sativum	Y	Caution	Y	None	PREGNANCY: Excessive use is not advisable due to potential emmenagogue and uterine-stimulating effects; standardized garlic preparations are believed not to have these effects. MALE FERTILITY: Traditionally viewed as an aphrodisiac, garlic can serve as a substitute for prescription male enhancement products due to its ability to sustain erections.
GINGER	Zingiber officinale	Caution	Caution	Y	None	PRECONCEPTION & PREGNANCY: Ginger is safe in culinary amounts or as part of herbal teas, but excessive use is not advisable due to potential emmenagogue and abortifacient effects.

PRE=PRECONCEPTION
PREG=PREGNANCY
BF=BREASTFEEDING

Pregnancy Safety Resource

PRE=PRECONCEPTION
PREG=PREGNANCY
BF=BREASTFEEDING

HERB	LATIN NAME	PRE	PREG	BF	ALTERNATIVE	ADDITIONAL NOTES
GINGKO	Gingko biloba	Y	Y	Caution	None	POSTPARTUM: Wait to use until postpartum bleeding has ceased, as the herb can act as a blood thinner that may promote blood flow. MALE FERTILITY: Ginkgo is beneficial for impotence as it enhances blood flow to the penile artery, sustaining erections without negatively affecting blood pressure.
GINSENG	Panax ginseng	Y	Y	Y	None	MALE FERTILITY: Traditionally believed to be an aphrodisiac, ginseng can be used as an alternative to prescription male enhancement products due to its ability to sustain erections.
GOAT'S RUE	Galega officinalis	Y	Y	Y	None	ETHNOBOTANY: Traditionally used in European herbal medicine for its potential to increase milk production in nursing mothers and manage blood sugar levels. PREGNANCY: Use with caution; can stimulate uterine contractions and may have emmenagogue effects. Best to avoid without medical supervision. LACTATION: Often used to support lactation;
GOJI BERRY	Lycium barbarum	Y	Caution	Y	Bilberry (Vaccinium myrtillus) for eye and antioxidant support.	ETHNOBOTANY: A key component of Traditional Chinese Medicine (TCM), goji berries are often used to nourish the body and support longevity. PRECONCEPTION: Provides antioxidants and supports overall health. PREGNANCY: Use cautiously due to potential blood pressure-lowering effects. LACTATION: Provides antioxidants.
GOLDENROD	Solidago virgauerea	Y	Y	Y	None	ETHNOBOTANY: Traditionally used in Native American medicine for various ailments, including urinary tract infections and respiratory issues. PRECONCEPTION: Generally considered safe; may support urinary health. PREGNANCY: Use with caution; some sources recommend avoiding high doses due to potential uterine stimulation. LACTATION: Generally considered safe; may help with lactation support and has mild anti-inflammatory properties.

Pregnancy Safety Resource

HERB	LATIN NAME	PRE	PREG	BF	ALTERNATIVE	ADDITIONAL NOTES
GOLDENSEAL	*Hydrastis canadensis*	Y	N	N	Marsh tea homeopathic, Shiitake, Elder	ETHNOBOTANY: Traditionally used by Native Americans for its medicinal properties, particularly for respiratory and digestive issues. PRECONCEPTION: Considered a uterine stimulant; use with caution. PREGNANCY & LACTATION: Recommended only for topical use.
GOTU KOLA	*Centella asiatica*	Y	Y	Y	None	ETHNOBOTANY: Widely used in traditional medicine in Asia for its cognitive and healing properties; often referred to as a "brain tonic." PREGNANCY: Generally considered safe in culinary amounts, but high doses should be avoided due to potential uterine stimulation. LACTATION: Considered safe in moderate amounts; may support lactation and enhance milk production.
GUARANA	*Paullinia cupana*	Caution	Caution	Caution	None	PRECONCEPTION: Guaranine, identical to caffeine, is extremely drying to cervical fluids and can burden the endocrine system, leading to hormonal imbalances. PREGNANCY: Guaranine crosses the placenta, potentially contributing to low birth weight, preterm birth, and birth defects. LACTATION: Guaranine appears in breast milk at half the level found in the mother's plasma and reduces the available iron supply in breast milk.
GUAVA	*Psidium guajava*	Y	Y	Y	Orange (Citrus sinensis) for a similar vitamin profile.	PRECONCEPTION: Supports immune function and provides essential vitamins. PREGNANCY: Rich in folate, crucial for fetal development. LACTATION: Provides vitamin C and aids in digestion. ETHNOBOTANY: Common in tropical regions, guava is used in culinary and medicinal contexts; guava leaves are valued for their antimicrobial properties.
HAWTHORN	*Crataegus spp.*	Y	Y	Y	None	MALE FERTILITY: An important circulatory tonic that supports fertility.

PRE=PRECONCEPTION
PREG=PREGNANCY
BF=BREASTFEEDING

Pregnancy Safety Resource

PRE=PRECONCEPTION
PREG=PREGNANCY
BF=BREASTFEEDING

HERB	LATIN NAME	PRE	PREG	BF	ALTERNATIVE	ADDITIONAL NOTES
HIBISCUS	*Hibiscus sabdariffa*	Y	Caution	Y	Rosehip (Rosa canina) for vitamin C and antioxidant support.	PREGNANCY: Excessive use in early pregnancy should be avoided due to potential emmenagogue and abortifacient effects.
HOLY BASIL	*Ocimum sanctum*	Y	Y	Y	None	ETHNOBOTANY: Revered in Ayurvedic medicine, known as "Tulsi," used for its adaptogenic properties and spiritual significance in Hindu culture. PRECONCEPTION: May help reduce stress and balance hormones; considered beneficial for reproductive health. PREGNANCY: Generally safe in culinary amounts; high doses should be avoided as they may have uterine stimulant effects. LACTATION: Believed to enhance milk production; safe when consumed in moderation.
HOREHOUND	*Marrubium vulgare*	Caution	N	Y	Elecampane, Mullein	PRECONCEPTION: Emmenagogue. PREGNANCY: Emmenagogue and abortifacient due to uterine stimulation.
HORSETAIL	*Equisetum spp.*	Y	Y	Caution	CALCIUM SUPPLEMENT: Oatstraw DIURETIC: Dandelion	LACTATION: Due to its high inorganic silica content, it is best to minimize use of this herb to prevent potential negative reactions in nursing mothers.
HYSSOP	*Hyssopus officinalis*	Y	Caution	Caution	Elecampane, Mullein	PRECONCEPTION: Emmenagogue. PREGNANCY: Emmenagogue and abortifacient.
HOREHOUND	*Marrubium vulgare*	Caution	N	Y	Elecampane, Mullein	PREGNANCY: Emmenagogue and abortifacient due to uterine stimulation.
JAMAICAN DOGWOOD	*Piscidia piscipula*	Y	N	N	Skullcap (Scutellaria lateriflora) for relaxation and pain relief.	ETHNOBOTANY: Traditionally used in Caribbean medicine for pain and insomnia. PRECONCEPTION: Used for pain relief and relaxation. PREGNANCY: Generally avoided due to strong sedative effects. LACTATION: Not recommended due to potential toxicity.

Pregnancy Safety Resource

PRE=PRECONCEPTION | PREG=PREGNANCY | BF=BREASTFEEDING

HERB	LATIN NAME	PRE	PREG	BF	ALTERNATIVE	ADDITIONAL NOTES
JUNIPER	*Juniperus communis*	Caution	N	Y	Goldenrod	PRECONCEPTION: Urinary tract irritant that may have a secondary effect as a uterine stimulant.
KAVA KAVA	*Piper methysticum*	Y	Caution	Caution	Lemon balm, Rose, Lavender	PREGNANCY: Pyrone in kava may cause loss of uterine tone. LACTATION: Kava is contraindicated for depression and is linked to liver toxicity, particularly with excessive dosage, alcoholism, or prescription drug use. Its safety is not conclusively established, and pyrones may pass into breast milk.
LADY'S MANTLE	*Alchemilla vulgaris*	Caution	Caution	Y	Blackberry Root	PRECONCEPTION & PREGNANCY: In some sources, the tonic nature of the herb is viewed as a possible uterine stimulant.
LAVENDER	*Lavendula angustifolia*	Y	Y	Y	None	PREGNANCY: Generally considered safe in culinary amounts; however, caution is advised due to potential hormonal effects. LACTATION: Considered safe in culinary amounts; high doses may affect milk production. PRECONCEPTION: May have mild effects on mood and stress relief. Note: Lavender is an endocrine disruptor and should not be used in high amounts, especially on prepubescent children, particularly boys.
LEMON BALM	*Melissa officinalis*	Caution	Caution	Y	FOR DEPRESSION/ANXIETY: Rose	PRECONCEPTION: Emmenagogue in therapeutic doses. PREGNANCY: Some recorded instances of use as an emmenagogue; however, it tends to inhibit thyroid and gonadotropic hormones. It is best used in non-therapeutic doses as a flavoring in herbal teas or food, not as an active herbal therapy during pregnancy.
LEMONGRASS	*Cymbopogon citratus*	Y	Caution	Y	Cramp Bark, Eucalyptus, Ginger for nausea	PREGNANCY: In therapeutic doses, lemongrass is reported to be an emmenagogue. Use only as a flavoring ingredient in culinary amounts during pregnancy.

Pregnancy Safety Resource

BF=BREASTFEEDING
PREG=PREGNANCY
PRE=PRECONCEPTION

HERB	LATIN NAME	PRE	PREG	BF	ALTERNATIVE	ADDITIONAL NOTES
LICORICE	*Glycyrrhiza glabra*	Caution	Caution	Caution	Borage	PRECONCEPTION & PREGNANCY: Licorice can be used as an emmenagogue. LACTATION: The concentration of glycyrrhetinic acid in the herb may cause unsafe retention of sodium and potassium in the nursing mother or child, which is especially dangerous for those with high blood pressure. MALE FERTILITY: Licorice is beneficial for men due to its ability to support adrenal function. Stress that weakens the adrenals is a common cause of sexual dysfunction, making this herb important for restoring vitality to the male reproductive system.
LOBELIA	*Lobelia inflate*	Caution	N	N	Elecampane, Wild Cherry Bark, Cramp Bark	PRECONCEPTION: Lobelia can potentially interfere with uterine tone and threaten fetal viability due to the toxicity of the alkaloid lobeline. LACTATION: In large doses, lobelia poses a potential toxin risk for the nursing infant; in smaller doses, it carries a risk of emesis. Lobeline, similar to nicotine, may transmit to the infant, leading to immediate changes in respiration and oxygen saturation, and may also affect a child's intelligence and behavioral development.
MACA	*Lepidium meyenii*	Y	Y	Y	Ashwagandha (Withania somnifera) for similar adaptogenic effects.	MALE FERTILITY: Maca is a nutritive tonic that supports male fertility.
MARSH-MALLOW	*Althea officinalis*	Y	Y	Y	None	PRECONCEPTION: Can be beneficial for mucosal health and digestive support. PREGNANCY: Generally safe and may support digestive health and soothe the gastrointestinal tract. LACTATION: Considered safe; may help with hydration and soothing throat discomfort.

HERB	LATIN NAME	PRE	PREG	BF	ALTERNATIVE	ADDITIONAL NOTES
MATE	Ilex paraguayensis	Caution	Caution	Caution	None	PRECONCEPTION: Caffeine is extremely drying to cervical fluids and places an unnecessary burden on the endocrine system, potentially leading to hormonal imbalance. PREGNANCY: Caffeine crosses the placenta and may contribute to low birth weight, preterm delivery, and birth defects. LACTATION: Caffeine appears in breast milk at half the concentration found in the mother's plasma and reduces the available iron supply in breast milk.
MEADOW-SWEET	Filipendula ulmaria	Y	Y	Y	None	PRECONCEPTION May support digestive health and has anti-inflammatory properties. PREGNANCY: Generally considered safe; may help relieve minor aches and pains. LACTATION: Usually safe, but excessive use should be avoided due to potential interactions with breastfeeding.
MILK THISTLE	Silybum marianum	Y	Y	Y	None	PRECONCEPTION: Supports liver function and detoxification; potentially beneficial for overall reproductive health. Pregnancy: Generally considered safe, but high doses should be avoided; consult a healthcare provider. Lactation: Safe for breastfeeding; may enhance milk production and support liver health.
MOTHERWORT	Leonurus cardianca	Caution	Caution	Y	ERRATIC HEART: Valerian	PRECONCEPTION: Emmenagogue. PREGNANCY: Excessive use should be avoided in early pregnancy to prevent miscarriage.

Pregnancy Safety Resource

PRE=PRECONCEPTION
PREG=PREGNANCY
BF=BREASTFEEDING

Pregnancy Safety Resource

PRE=PRECONCEPTION
PREG=PREGNANCY
BF=BREASTFEEDING

HERB	LATIN NAME	PRE	PREG	BF	ALTERNATIVE	ADDITIONAL NOTES
MORINGA	Moringa oleifera	Y	Y	Y	Alfalfa (Medicago sativa) for similar nutritional benefits.	ETHNOBOTANY: Known as the "miracle tree," it is widely used in tropical countries for its medicinal and nutritional benefits. PREGNANCY: Avoid seeds. LACTATION: Enhances milk production and provides vital nutrients to both mother and baby.
MUGWORT	Artemesia vulgare	Caution	N	N	Gentian, Dandelion Root, Artichoke	PREGNANCY: Uterine stimulant. LACTATION: Thujone in mugwort can negatively affect breast milk. Avoid essential oils or alcoholic extracts and use sparingly. Mugwort's bitterness may aid in weaning; reduce usage if the baby pulls away.
MUIRA PUAMA	Ptychopetalum olacoides	Y	Y	Y	None	
MULLEIN	Verbascum thapsus	Y	Y	Y	None	PRECONCEPTION: Supports respiratory and lung health, potentially beneficial for overall wellness. PREGNANCY: Generally considered safe; used for respiratory support. LACTATION: Generally safe; may support respiratory health in nursing mothers and infants.
MUSHROOM	look at notes for types	Y	Y	Y	None	Turkey Tail, Shiitake, Reishi, Maitake, Chaga, Cordyceps all safe in all conditions.
MYRRH	Commiphora myrrha	Caution	Caution	Y	None	PRECONCEPTION: Can cause contractions. PREGNANCY: Can act as a uterine stimulant, potentially causing contractions. Limit use to occasional tooth product additives during pregnancy.
OATS	Milky Oats/Oat Tops/Oatstraw	Y	Y	Y	None	MALE FERTILITY: Milky oats are particularly beneficial when male impotence is linked to stress.
OREGON GRAPE ROOT	Mahonia aquifolium	Y	N	N	Marsh tea homeopathic, Shiitake, Elder	PREGNANCY: Berberine, an alkaloid, is a mild toxin with depressant effects on the heart and lungs and may act as a uterine stimulant at certain doses. LACTATION: Berberine, a mild toxin, can depress heart and lung function and may stimulate the uterus at certain doses. It could be especially problematic if the baby has jaundice.
OSHA	Ligusticum porter	Caution	N	Y	None	PRECONCEPTION & PREGNANCY: Emmenagogue.

HERB	LATIN NAME	PRE	PREG	BF	ALTERNATIVE	ADDITIONAL NOTES
PAPAYA	*Carica papaya*	Y	Y	Y	Mango (Mangifera indica) for a similar nutrient profile.	PREGNANCY: Avoid unripe papaya due to potential uterine contractions. LACTATION: Aids in digestion and milk production.
PAPAYA LEAF	*Carica papaya*	Y	Caution	Caution	Dandelion Leaf (Taraxacum officinale): Supports digestive health and immune function.	ETHNOBOTANY: In tropical regions, papaya is widely used for its digestive and anti-inflammatory properties. PREGNANCY: Used for low platelets; use with caution during pregnancy.
PARSLEY	*Petroselinum crispum*	Caution	Caution	Caution	None	ROOT USE: Not safe during pregnancy; safe for preconception and breastfeeding. PRECONCEPTION & PREGNANCY (Aerial Portions): Use sparingly as a culinary herb. In therapeutic doses, it can act as an emmenagogue. PREGNANCY (Root): Parsley root is an emmenagogue, abortifacient, and uterine stimulant. LACTATION (Aerial Portions): May reduce milk volume with significant intake. Safe in food unless overly sensitive; monitor milk flow and avoid parsley-heavy foods.
PARTRIDGE-BERRY	*Mitchella repens*	Y	Y	Y	None	PRECONCEPTION: Used as a tonic for reproductive health, potentially beneficial for preparing the body for pregnancy. PREGNANCY: Traditionally used to support uterine health and facilitate labor; however, consult a healthcare provider before use. LACTATION: Considered safe; may support milk production and overall maternal health.
PASSION-FLOWER	*Passiflora incarnata*	Y	Caution	Y	Chamomile, Skullcap, Valerian	PREGNANCY: The herb may act as a uterine stimulant due to the presence of the alkaloids harman and harmaline.

Pregnancy Safety Resource

PRE=PRECONCEPTION
PREG=PREGNANCY
BF=BREASTFEEDING

Pregnancy Safety Resource

HERB	LATIN NAME	PRE	PREG	BF	ALTERNATIVE	ADDITIONAL NOTES
PAU D'ARCO	Tabebuia impetiginosa	Y	Y	Y	None	PRECONCEPTION: Traditionally used for its potential immune-supportive properties; however, high doses should be avoided. PREGNANCY: Use cautiously; may stimulate uterine contractions in high doses. LACTATION: Safety during breastfeeding is not well established; consult a healthcare provider before use.
PEACH	Prunus persica	Caution	N	N	None	BARK/LEAF: Okay for all conditions. PRECONCEPTION (SEED): Peach pits can act as an emmenagogue. PREGNANCY (SEED): A high concentration of cyanogenic glycosides makes this part of the plant potentially deadly, as well as an emmenagogue and abortifacient. Pregnancy is not the time to address pelvic stagnation. LACTATION (SEED): A high concentration of cyanogenic glycosides makes this part of the plant potentially deadly.
PENNYROYAL	Hedeoma pulegoides	Caution	Caution	Y	None	PRECONCEPTION & PREGNANCY: Well-known emmenagogue and abortifacient
PEONY	Paeonia officinalis	Y	Caution	Y	PAIN: Rosemary SWELLING: Poultice of Yarrow	PREGNANCY: Excessive use should be avoided in early pregnancy, as it acts as an emmenagogue.
PEPPERMINT	Mentha piperita	Y	Caution	Y	None	PREGNANCY (LEAVES): Excessive use of leaves should be avoided early in pregnancy, as volatile oils can cross the placenta and act as an emmenagogue. PREGNANCY (ESSENTIAL OIL): Believed to be an emmenagogue; essential oil should not be used during pregnancy. LACTATION (ESSENTIAL OIL): Use essential oil with caution, as inhalation by infants can cause adverse nervous system reactions.
PINE	Pinus spp.	Caution	N	Y	Elecampane, Mullein	PRECONCEPTION: Abortifacient qualities. PREGNANCY: Abortifacient qualities.

PRE=PRECONCEPTION PREG=PREGNANCY BF=BREASTFEEDING

Pregnancy Safety Resource

HERB	LATIN NAME	PRE	PREG	BF	ALTERNATIVE	ADDITIONAL NOTES
PLANTAIN	*Plantago spp.*	Y	Y	Y	None	PREGNANCY: Generally safe and used for digestive support; consult a healthcare provider for therapeutic use. LACTATION: Considered safe; may support lactation and digestive health. PRECONCEPTION: Used traditionally for its anti-inflammatory and wound-healing properties.
PLEURISY ROOT	*Asclepias tuberosa*	Y	N	N	Elecampane, Mullein	PREGNANCY & LACTATION: Side effects of cardiac glycosides may include uterine stimulation and estrogenic activity.
POKE ROOT	*Phytolacca americana*	Caution	N	Caution	DISSOLVE LUMPS IN BREAST TISSUE WITH BREASTFEEDING: Poultice of Tumeric	PRECONCEPTION: Lectins in all parts of poke are toxic and can lead to clumping of red blood cells and rapid, uncontrolled cell growth. PREGNANCY: The lectins in all parts of poke are toxic and can lead to clumping of red blood cells and rapid, uncontrolled cell growth. LACTATION: Poke root is often used in breast balm and for breast self-exams and routine massage, but it may have an undesired laxative effect in nursing infants.
POMEGRANATE	*Punica granatum*	N	N	N	Pumpkin Seeds, Garlic, Black Walnut Hull	PRECONCEPTION, PREGNANCY, AND LACTATION: Pomegranate bark is harsh, purgative, and can act as an emmenagogue and uterine stimulant.
RED CLOVER	*Trifolium pratense*	Y	Caution	Y	Dandelion Root, Burdock	PREGNANCY: Red clover contains natural coumarins, which are a class of blood thinners. This action appears to be mild and has not caused problems in animals or humans. While the anticoagulant nature of this herb is only suspected, it's important for women to be mindful when using it during pregnancy, as blood volume changes frequently during this time.

PRE=PRECONCEPTION
PREG=PREGNANCY
BF=BREASTFEEDING

Pregnancy Safety Resource

PRE=PRECONCEPTION
PREG=PREGNANCY
BF=BREASTFEEDING

HERB	LATIN NAME	PRE	PREG	BF	ALTERNATIVE	ADDITIONAL NOTES
RED RASPBERRY	*Rubus idaeus*	Y	Y	Y	None	MALE FERTILITY: Red raspberry is considered an important tonic for the male reproductive system, similar to its benefits for females.
RHUBARB	*Rheum palmatum*	N	N	Caution	Dandelion Root, Yellow Dock Root	PRECONCEPTION: Rhubarb is a uterine stimulant with potential mutagens that are not advisable to be present in pre-pregnancy tissues. PREGNANCY: Rhubarb is a uterine stimulant with strong downward energy and potential mutagenic effects due to anthraquinones. It also carries a risk of kidney damage due to its high oxalate content. LACTATION: As anthraquinones are partially excreted in milk, rhubarb may have a laxative effect on infants and could pass along the genotoxins emodin and aloe-emodin.
ROMAN CHAMOMILE	*Chamaemelum nobile*	Caution	Caution	Y	German chamomile	PRECONCEPTION & PREGNANCY: Extremely high doses can act as an emmenagogue and abortifacient.
ROSE	*Rosa spp.*	Y	Y	Y	None	PRECONCEPTION: Known for its toning properties and is often used in herbal preparations for reproductive health. PREGNANCY: Generally safe; used for its calming properties and to support emotional well-being. LACTATION: Safe for use; may help with milk production and provide soothing effects.

HERB	LATIN NAME	PRE	PREG	BF	ALTERNATIVE	ADDITIONAL NOTES
ROSEMARY	*Rosmarinus officinalis*	Caution	Caution	Y	None	PRECONCEPTION: Rosemary acts as an emmenagogue in therapeutic doses. PREGNANCY: Therapeutic doses of rosemary are not appropriate during pregnancy due to potential emmenagogue and abortifacient effects; however, occasional use in herbal tea or as a seasoning is acceptable.
RUE	*Ruta graveolens*	Caution	N	Y	None	PRECONCEPTION: Emmenagogue. PREGNANCY: Emmenagogue that may cause contractions.
SAGE	*Salvia officinalis*	Y	Caution	Caution	SORE THROAT: Pau D'arco, Thyme	NO USE of essential oil/alcoholic extract in any condition. PRECONCEPTION & PREGNANCY (Essential Oil/Alcoholic Extract Use): Internal use can act as an emmenagogue and abortifacient. PREGNANCY (Leaf Use): Due to thujone content, high doses of tea or excessive use can be an emmenagogue or abortifacient. LACTATION (Leaf Use): Sage is known as an anti-galactagogue and may reduce milk supply. LACTATION (Essential Oil/Alcoholic Extract Use): Internal use can negatively affect the breastfeeding baby due to thujone content.
SENNA	*Cassia spp.*	N	N	N	Dandelion Root, Yellow Dock Root	PRECONCEPTION: Use with caution; should be avoided in therapeutic doses due to potential uterine stimulation. PREGNANCY: Generally not recommended due to its strong laxative effects, which can stimulate uterine contractions. LACTATION: Caution advised; may pass into breast milk and cause diarrhea in nursing infants.

Pregnancy Safety Resource

PRE=PRECONCEPTION
PREG=PREGNANCY
BF=BREASTFEEDING

Pregnancy Safety Resource

PRE=PRECONCEPTION
PREG=PREGNANCY
BF=BREASTFEEDING

HERB	LATIN NAME	PRE	PREG	BF	ALTERNATIVE	ADDITIONAL NOTES
SHATAVARI	*Asparagus racemosus*	Y	Y	Y	None	PRECONCEPTION: Supports fertility and reproductive health; often recommended for women trying to conceive. PREGNANCY: Considered safe; traditionally used to support reproductive health and hormonal balance. LACTATION: Promotes lactation and is often used as a galactagogue.
SHEPHERD'S PURSE	*Capsella bursa-pastoris*	Caution	N	Caution	Plantain	PRECONCEPTION: Consume this herb only when cooked; high levels of oxalic acid can bind to calcium, leading to deficiencies. PREGNANCY: Shepherd's Purse contains high amounts of oxalic acid, which can potentially damage developing kidneys; it is also a known emmenagogue and abortifacient. LACTATION: Consume this herb only when cooked; high levels of oxalic acid can bind to calcium, leading to deficiencies.
SKULLCAP	*Scutellaria lateriflora*	Y	Y	Y	None	PRECONCEPTION: Traditionally used for stress relief and nervous system support; caution advised due to possible uterine effects.
SLIPPERY ELM	*Ulmus rubra*	Y	Y	Y	None	PRECONCEPTION: Used for its soothing properties and to support digestive health; generally regarded as safe in moderation. Pregnancy: Generally considered safe in food amounts; used for digestive support. LACTATION: Considered safe; may help soothe gastrointestinal issues in nursing mothers.
SOURSOP	*Annona muricata*	Y	Use in culinary amount	Y	None	ETHNOBOTANY: Soursop leaves are traditionally used in Caribbean and South American herbal medicine for their various health benefits.

HERB	LATIN NAME	PRE	PREG	BF	ALTERNATIVE	ADDITIONAL NOTES
SOURSOP LEAF	*Annona muricata*	Y	Caution	Y	Soursop fruit in culinary amount	PREGNANCY: Use with caution; some sources recommend avoiding this herb due to its strong bioactive compounds.
SPEARMINT	*Mentha spicata*	Y	Y	Y	None	PRECONCEPTION: Used for digestive support; generally regarded as safe in moderate amounts. PREGNANCY: Generally considered safe in culinary amounts; may help with digestion and nausea. LACTATION: Considered safe; may support digestion and milk production.
SPIRULINA	*Arthrospira platensis*	Y	Y	Y	None	PRECONCEPTION: Nutrient-dense; may support overall health and vitality when trying to conceive. PREGNANCY: Considered safe in moderate amounts; rich in nutrients beneficial for pregnant women. LACTATION: Generally safe; may support nutrition and energy levels for nursing mothers.
ST. JOHN'S WORT	*Hypericum perforatum*	Y	N	Caution	ANXIETY & DEPRESSION: Lavender, Rose, Lemon Balm, Chamomile	PREGNANCY: Known as an emmenagogue and abortifacient. LACTATION: If a nursing child is being treated for jaundice, this herb may increase sensitivity to UV light; avoid using it until treatments are completed.
Tamarind	*Tamarindus indica*	Y	Use in culinary amount	Y	Prunes (Prunus domestica) for similar digestive support.	ETHNOBOTANY: Widely utilized in African, Asian, and Latin American cuisines and traditional medicine. PRECONCEPTION: Used as a natural laxative. PREGNANCY: Can be used in moderation to support digestion and relieve constipation.

Pregnancy Safety Resource

PRE=PRECONCEPTION
PREG=PREGNANCY
BF=BREASTFEEDING

Pregnancy Safety Resource

BF=BREASTFEEDING
PREG=PREGNANCY
PRE=PRECONCEPTION

HERB	LATIN NAME	PRE	PREG	BF	ALTERNATIVE	ADDITIONAL NOTES
Tansy	*Tanacetum vulgar*	Caution	N	N	Pumpkin Seeds, Garlic, Black Walnut Hull	PRECONCEPTION: Emmenagogue. PREGNANCY: While the essential oil of tansy is most problematic, tansy itself is too variable in its constituent levels to say it is safe as a tea during pregnancy. It is best avoided in favor of another herb during this time. Empirical evidence shows tansy to be a uterine stimulant, emmenagogue, and abortifacient with the potential to cause birth defects. LACTATION: Thujone is a compound that, when taken in incorrect doses, can be toxic to both mother and infant.
TOBACCO	*Nicotiana tabacum*	N	N	N	None	PRECONCEPTION & PREGNANCY: Tobacco is known to contribute to low birth weights, birth defects, miscarriage, and preterm labor. LACTATION: Avoid ingestion of tobacco in any form; it is known to result in a diminished milk supply. The excretion of nicotine in breast milk has been shown to cause immediate changes in respiration and oxygen saturation in the breastfeeding infant. It is also believed that it may alter a child's intelligence and behavioral development, and the inhalation of secondhand smoke is thought to increase future chances for lung cancer.
TUMERIC	*Curcuma longa*	Caution	Caution	Y	Bitter Orange, Chamomile, Meadowsweet, Elder	PRECONCEPTION: Avoid therapeutic doses while trying to become pregnant, as turmeric can act as an emmenagogue. PREGNANCY: Although turmeric is an effective therapy for many imbalances, at therapeutic doses during pregnancy it can act as an emmenagogue or abortifacient. If used in food or in tea, it is relatively safe.
VALERIAN	*Valeriana officinalis*	Y	Y	Y	None	PRECONCEPTION : Traditionally used to support relaxation and reduce stress, which may benefit fertility. PREGNANCY: Use cautiously; may have sedative effects. Limited studies on safety. LACTATION: Avoid high doses; may affect nursing infants' sleep patterns.

Pregnancy Safety Resource

HERB	LATIN NAME	PRE	PREG	BF	ALTERNATIVE	ADDITIONAL NOTES
WILD CHERRY	Prunus serotina	Caution	Caution	Y	Elecampane, Cramp Bark	PRECONCEPTION & PREGNANCY: The presence of cyanogenic glycosides (prunasin) is believed to be teratogenic when taken in excessive doses or for prolonged periods.
WILD YAM	Dioscorea villosa	Y	Caution	Y	LIVER STAGNATION: Dandelion Root	PREGNANCY: Wild yam has been noted to act as a uterine stimulant.
YARROW	Achillea millefolium	Caution	Caution	Caution	None	Essential Oil/Alcoholic Extract Use: No use in any condition.
YELLOW DOCK	Rumex crispus	Y	Y	Y	None	PREGNANCY: Use with caution; high oxalate content may affect calcium absorption. LACTATION: Considered safe in moderation; may have a mild laxative effect. PRECONCEPTION: Traditionally used for digestive health and to support nutrient absorption.
YERBA MATE	Ilex paraguariensis	Y	Caution	Caution	Green tea (Camellia sinensis) for a milder caffeine boost.	PREGNANCY & LACTATION: Contains caffeine. Use in moderation; excessive use can lead to sleep disturbances.
YERBA SANTA	Eriodictyon californicum	Y	Caution	Y	Mullein (Verbascum thapsus) for respiratory support.	ETHNOBOTANY: Known as "holy herb," native to the southwestern United States and Mexico, traditionally used by indigenous peoples for respiratory conditions. PREGNANCY: Used cautiously for respiratory issues.

PRE=PRECONCEPTION
PREG=PREGNANCY
BF=BREASTFEEDING

REFERENCES

- American College of Nurse-Midwives. (2021). Incorporating cultural traditions and practices in women's health care. ACNM Position Statement.
- Arizpe, L. (1997). Childbirth in Mexico: inculturation or medicalization? In R. Davis-Floyd & C. F. Sargent (Eds.), Childbirth and authoritative knowledge: Cross-Cultural perspectives (pp. 180-198). University of California Press. https://doi.org/10.1525/9780520918733
- Balasubramanian, H., et al. (2018). Empathy, connectedness, and organizational culture drive positive patient experience. Journal of Healthcare Management, 63(5), 347-360.
- Beck C. T. (2023). Experiences of postpartum depression in women of color. MCN. The American Journal of Maternal Child Nursing, 48(2), 88–95. https://doi.org/10.1097/NMC.0000000000000889
- Bodnar-Deren, S., Benn, E. K. T., Balbierz, A., et al. (2017). Stigma and postpartum depression treatment acceptability among black and white women in the first six-months postpartum. Matern Child Health J(21), 1457–1468. doi: 10.1007/s10995-017-2263-6.
- Cohen, M., Harvey, N., & Lipton, B. (2018). Postpartum massage and pelvic floor function: a pilot study. Journal of Alternative and Complementary Medicine, 24(2), 123-136. doi: 10.1089/acm.2017.0084
- Combs, Dawn. Conceiving Healthy Babies: An Herbal Guide to Supporting Conception and Pregnancy. Herbal Media Group, 2017.
- Covert, B. (2021, July 27). The unseen costs of parental leave. The New York Times. https://www.nytimes.com/2021/07/27/opinion/parental-leave.html
- Brodsky, S. (2008). Where have all the midwives gone. The Journal Of Perinatal Education, Fall, 48-51. https://www.ncbi.nlm.nih.gov/pmc/articles/PMC2582410/
- Bureau of Labor Statistics. (2021). Paid family leave in the United States. Monthly Labor Review, 144(6). https://www.bls.gov/opub/mlr/2021/article/paid-family-leave-in-the-united-states.htm
- Celtic Medical Treatments. (n.d.). Royal College of Physicians of Edinburgh. www.rcpe.ac.uk/heritage/celtic-medical-treatments#:~:text=Infusion%20of%20wild%20garlic%20was,to%20the%20island%20of%20Taransay
- Centers for Disease Control and Prevention. (2020, October 28). Pregnancy Mortality Surveillance System. CDC. www.cdc.gov/reproductivehealth/maternal-mortality/pregnancy-mortality-surveillance-system.htm
- Chien, L.-Y., Tai, C.-J., Ko, Y.-L., Huang, C.-H., & Sheu, S.-J. (2006). Adherence to "Doing-the-month" practices is associated with fewer physical and depressive symptoms among postpartum women in Taiwan. Research in Nursing & Health, 29(4), 374-383. doi: 10.1002/nur.20154
- Cultural appropriation: A guide for non-Indigenous people. (2017). CBC News Indigenous. https://www.cbc.ca/news/indigenous/cultural-appropriation-a-guide-for-non-indigenous-people-1.4046304
- Cohen, M., Harvey, N., & Lipton, B. (2018). Postpartum massage and pelvic floor function: A pilot study. Journal of Alternative and Complementary Medicine, 24(2), 123-136. doi: 10.1089/acm.2017.0084
- Covert, B. (2021, July 27). The unseen costs of parental leave. The New York Times. https://www.nytimes.com/2021/07/27/opinion/parental-leave.html
- Creanga, A. A., et al. (2014, May). Racial and ethnic disparities in severe maternal morbidity: a multistate analysis, 2008-2010. American Journal of Obstetrics and Gynecology, 210(5), 435.e1-435.e8. doi: https://doi.org/10.1016/j.ajog.2013.11.039
- Dishman, L. (2015, December 10). What Marissa Mayer's maternity leave decision means for working parents at Yahoo. Fast Company. https://www.fastcompany.com/3054512/what-marissa-mayers-maternity-leave-decision-means-for-working-parents-at-yahoo
- Encyclopædia Britannica. (2022, January 12). Revolution. https://www.britannica.com/topic/revolution-politics
- Galactagogues Information Sheet [PDF]. Sarah Oakley Lactation. https://sarahoakleylactation.co.uk/wp-content/uploads/2021/03/Galactagogues-info-sheet.pdf
- Gladstar, Rosemary. Healing for Women: An Herbal Guide to Balancing Hormones and Supporting Health. Storey Publishing, 2012.
- Graham, L., et al. (2013). Indigenous women's views on maternity care in rural British Columbia. Journal of Aboriginal Health, 9(2), 18-27.

- Green, D. M., Duffee, K., & May, M. (2019). The use of rebozo technique in pregnancy, labor, and postpartum. Journal of Perinatal Education, 28(2), 95-104. doi: 10.1891/1058-1243.28.2.95
- Grimes, R. L. (2000). Deeply into the bone: re-inventing rites of passage. University of California Press. doi: https://doi.org/10.1086/491157
- Hanley, M. R. L., & Bottorff, J. L. (2013). Postpartum practices among indigenous women in Canada: a systematic review. Journal of Obstetric, Gynecologic, and Neonatal Nursing, 42(6), 732-743. doi: 10.1111/1552-6909.12258
- Heese, A. (2023, January 17). Personal interview.
- Heese, A. (2017). Postpartum care in Australia: what women receive, what they want and what they need. Women and birth, 30(5), e202-e207. doi: 10.1016/j.wombi.2017.03.001
- Hollowell, J., Puddicombe, D., Rowe, R., Linsell, L., Hardy, P., Stewart, M., ... & Newburn, M. (2011). The Birthplace national prospective cohort study: perinatal and maternal outcomes by planned place of birth. Birthplace in England research programme. Final report part 4. NIHR service delivery and organisation programme.
- Hou, W.-H., et al. (2013). Biochemical and physiological changes following massage therapy: a review. Journal of Alternative and Complementary Medicine, 19(4), 270-280. doi: 10.1089/acm.2012.0058
- How to support indigenous communities: a guide for Canadians. (2021). CBC News Indigenous. https://www.cbc.ca/news/indigenous/how-to-support-indigenous-communities-1.5837762
- International Labour Organization (ILO) – Maternity protection database. https://www.ilo.org/dyn/travail/travmain.showYear?p_lang=en&p_jalon=PAY&p_nyear=2018&p_jetter=P&p_pay_cat=3
- Iverson, C., et al. (2018). Belly binding in a culturally diverse postpartum population. Journal of Alternative and Complementary Medicine, 24(10), 990-996. doi: 10.1089/acm.2018.0147
- Johns Hopkins Center for Communication Programs. (2021). Maternal mortality: Black mamas matter. Published 17 May 2021. https://ccp.jhu.edu/2021/05/17/maternal-mortality-black-mamas-race-momnibus/
- Jomeen, J., & Redshaw, M. (2013). Ethnic minority women's experience of maternity services in England. Ethnicity & Health, 18(3), 280-296. doi: 10.1080/13557858.2012.730608 https://www.tandfonline.com/doi/abs/10.1080/13557858.2012.730608
- Jones, S., Smith, M., & Johnson, L. (2014). Herbal remedies used by southern Black midwives: a descriptive study. Journal of Transcultural Nursing, 25(2), 174-182. doi: 10.1177/1043659613485422
- Jordan, B. (2017). Redefining the role of African American midwives in the United States. Journal of Transcultural Nursing, 28(6), 622-630. doi: 10.1177/1043659616687082
- Kaiser Family Foundation. (n.d.). Racial disparities in maternal and infant health: current status and efforts to address them. https://www.kff.org/racial-equity-and-health-policy/issue-brief/racial-disparities-in-maternal-and-infant-health-current-status-and-efforts-to-address-them/
- Katz Rothman, B., et al. (2015). Sustaining a traditional postpartum practice in a hospital setting. Journal of Obstetric, Gynecologic & Neonatal Nursing, 44(4), 508-517.
- Keefe, R. H., Brownstein-Evans, C., & Polmanteer, R. R. (2016). "I find peace there": how faith, church, and spirituality help mothers of colour cope with postpartum depression. Mental Health, Religion & Culture, 19(7), 722-733. doi: 10.1080/13674676.2016.1244663
- Kennedy, H. (2017). The risks of cesarean delivery for maternal and infant health. Seminars in Perinatology, 41(5), a283-287. doi: 10.1053/j.semperi.2017.05.007
- Khorsandi, M., et al. (2017). The effect of massage therapy on postpartum physiological and psychological well-being. Journal of Obstetrics and Gynaecology Research, 43(9), 1370-1377. doi: 10.1111/jog.13362
- Kildea, S. (2016). Wahakura: An indigenous child health intervention in New Zealand. The Lancet, 387(10024), 2528-2529. doi: 10.1016/S0140-6736(16)30729-6
- Kim, M. Y., et al. (2018). Korean maternity practices: an integrative review. Women and Birth, 31(5), e305-e313. doi: 10.1016/j.wombi.2017.12.004
- Kohn, M. A., & Lafreniere, D. (2017). Integrating complementary and alternative medicine with conventional healthcare: a review of the current evidence. International Journal of Behavioral Medicine, 24(6), 817-828.
- Langer, A., & Upreti, M. (2000). The impact of medical interventions on women's reproductive health and rights: a case study of Indigenous women in Mexico. Health and Human Rights Journal, 5(2), 86-108.
- Langer, A., et al. (2017). Why are there such high rates of cesarean delivery in Latin America? The Lancet, 389(10077), 587-599. doi: 10.1016/s0140-6736(16)31598-5

- Lavallee, L. F., et al. (2013). Postpartum health of Aboriginal women in Canada. Journal of Obstetric, Gynecologic, and Neonatal Nursing, 42(1), 24-36. doi: 10.1111/j.1552-6909.2012.01417.x
- LeCompte-Mastenbrook, J., et al. (2020). Improving the health of Native American women through traditional practices. Journal of Obstetric, Gynecologic & Neonatal Nursing, 49(2), 180-190.
- Linares, P. A. (2011). Honoring Indigenous women: the integration of traditional Native American practices in contemporary maternity care. Journal of Obstetric, Gynecologic & Neonatal Nursing, 40(3), 335-344.
- Lowe, J., et al. (2017). Integrating complementary and alternative medicine into conventional healthcare: a systematic review of clinical trials. International Journal of Clinical Practice, 71(11). doi: 10.1111/ijcp.12988
- Malcoe, L. H., & Bruce, N. (2019). Culture-based interventions and maternal health outcomes among Indigenous women in the United States: a systematic review. Health Equity, 3(1), 238-248. doi: 10.1089/heq.2019.0005
- Mayberry, L. J., Affonso, D. D., Shibuya, J. M., & Clemmens, D. M. (1999). Integrating cultural values, beliefs, and customs into pregnancy and postpartum care: lessons learned from a Hawaiian public health nursing project. The Journal of Perinatal & Neonatal Nursing, 13(1), 15-26.
- MBRRACE-UK Perinatal mortality surveillance. (n.d.). deprivation and ethnicity. TIMMS. https://timms.le.ac.uk/mbrrace-uk-perinatal-mortality/surveillance/#deprivation-and-ethnicity
- McDonald, B., et al. (2010). Indigenous women's health research and the cultural safety lens: a reciprocal relationship. Journal of Obstetric, Gynecologic, and Neonatal Nursing, 39(6), 680-685. doi: 10.1111/j.1552-6909.2010.01171.x
- McLeod, K., & Johnston, M. (2017). Integrating Indigenous birthing practices into western maternity care services. International Journal of Childbirth Education, 32(4), 14-18.
- Miller, A. R., Phillips, E., Alvarez, R. A., & Segura-Hernandez, L. (2021). The rebozo technique: a comprehensive review. Journal of Obstetric, Gynecologic & Neonatal Nursing, 50(4), 424-437. doi: 10.1016/j.jogn.2021.03.005
- Mitchell, Ross. Celtic medical treatments. (n.d.). Royal College of Physicians of Edinburgh. www.rcpe.ac.uk/heritage/celtic-medical-treatments#:~:text=Infusion%20of%20wild%20garlic%20was,to%20the%20island%20of%20Taransay
- Moritz, T., et al. (2020). Herbal remedies for postpartum bleeding and iron deficiency anemia: a systematic review. Journal of Midwifery & Women's Health, 65(2), 174-186. doi: 10.1111/jmwh.13004
- National partnership for women and families. (2019). Expecting better: A State-by-State Analysis of Laws That Help Expecting and New Parents. https://www.nationalpartnership.org/our-work/resources/economic-justice/expecting-better-2019.pdf
- Native Land Digital. (2021). Indigenous protocol guidelines. https://native-land.ca/protocols/
- Park, Y. L., & Canaway, R. (2019). Integrating traditional and complementary medicine with... Taylor and Francis. www.tandfonline.com/doi/full/10.1080/23288604.2018.1539058
- Rodriguez, T. (2018, Apr 18). Indigenous midwives in Mexico: bridging western and indigenous medicine. Sapiens. https://www.sapiens.org/biology/indigenous-midwives-mexico/
- Romer, A. L., et al. (2017). Closing the bones: an exploration of an Indigenous postpartum tradition. Journal of Perinatal Education, 26(1), 16-24. doi: 10.1891/1058-1243.26.1.16
- Rothman, B. K. (2005). The medicalization of childbirth. American Journal of Public Health, 95(8), 1358-1364.
- Savadogo, L. G., Kpozehouen, A., Bako, A. R., Wounangnon, G. M., Djigma, F. W., Soubeiga, S. T., ... & Simpore, J. (2023). Factors associated with intimate partner violence during pregnancy among women attending antenatal care in health facilities in Bobo-Dioulasso city, Burkina Faso: a cross-sectional study. BMC pregnancy and childbirth, 23(1), 1-10. https://doi.org/10.1186/s12884-023-05547-z
- Smith, J., et al. (2012). The effects of postpartum massage on maternal recovery. Journal of Midwifery and Women's Health, 57(5), 469-474. doi: 10.1111/j.1542-2011.2012.00197.x
- Stoll, K., & Hall, W. A. (2013). Walking the talk: the importance of aligning prenatal care with contemporary women's lives. Journal of Obstetrics and Gynaecology Canada, 35(3), 277-284.
- Thompson, J. (2005). Mother-roasting: a traditional postpartum health practice. Journal of Obstetric, Gynecologic, & Neonatal Nursing, 34(6), 713-722. doi: 10.1177/0884217505281747
- Topp, S. (2018). Indigenous pregnancy and birthing practices: an evidence scan. Women and Birth, 31(2), e77-e85. doi: 10.1016/j.wombi.2017.08.003
- Toulouse, P. R. (2010). Cultural safety and its importance for Ontario first nations: meaning and application for cultural competence. Journal of Aboriginal Health, 6(2), 22-31.

- Toulouse, P. R. (2010). Cultural safety and its importance for Ontario first nations: meaning and application for cultural competence. Journal of Aboriginal Health, 6(2), 22-31.
- Turocy, P. S., et al. (2019). The effects of postpartum abdominal binders on women's health outcomes. Journal of Alternative and Complementary Medicine, 25(1), 26-32. doi: 10.1089/acm.2017.0386
- UAE government portal. (n.d.) https://u.ae/en/information-and-services/jobs/working-maternity-and-childcare-leave
- U.S. department of labor. (n.d.) https://www.dol.gov/agencies/whd/fmla
- Wax, J. R., et al. (2010). Maternal and newborn outcomes in elective cesarean deliveries. Obstetrics & Gynecology, 115(3), 717-726. doi:10.1097/AOG.0b013e3181d559e0
- Weed, Susun. Wise Woman Herbal for the Childbearing Year. Ash Tree Publishing, 2002.
- Xygalatas, D. (2018). Ritual: how seemingly senseless acts make life worth living. Pantheon Books.
- Yamada, S., et al. (2019). Cultural safety training for healthcare providers on First Nations reserves in Canada: an interventional study. International Journal of Nursing Studies, 91, 1-9.
- Yates, S. R. (2012). African American women and the medicalization of childbirth in America: historical overview. Journal of African American Studies, 16(4), 579-597.
- Yee, L. M., et al. (2017). Epidural analgesia in normal labor. Obstetrics & Gynecology, 129(4), 675-680. doi:10.1097/AOG.
- Zahra Khojastehfard; Hamideh Yazdimoghaddam; Mahbubeh Abdollahi; Fatemeh Zahra Karimi. "Effect of Herbal Medicines on Postpartum Hemorrhage: A Systematic Review and Meta-Analysis", Evidence Based Care, 11, 1, 2021, 62-74. doi: 10.22038/ebcj.2021.58054.2513
- Zeng, M., Gong, A., & Wu, Z. (2022). Paroxetine combined with traditional Chinese medicine prescriptions in the treatment of postpartum depression: a systematic review of randomized controlled trials. Frontiers in Neuroendocrinology, 67, 101019. https://doi.org/10.1016/j.yfrne.2022.101019
- Zhang, X., Zuo, X., Matheï, C. et al. Impact of a postpartum care rehabilitation program to prevent postpartum depression at a secondary municipal hospital in Qingdao China: a cross-sectional study. BMC pregnancy childbirth 23, 239 (2023). https://doi.org/10.1186/s12884-023-05547-z

A

Aboriginal Traditions 137
Abortifacients 49, 52, 58
Adaptogens 54, 66, 67, 103, 105, 107
Affirmations 64
African Diaspora Traditions 139
African Traditions 138
Alfalfa (Medicago sativa) 54,65, 112, 119, 123
Alkaloids 49, 57, 58
Aloe (Aloe vera) 49, 58, 65, 70
Amaranth (Amaranthus spp.) 103
Ancient Egyptian Traditions 138
Anemia 69, 107
Angelica (Angelica archangelica) 49, 50
Anise (Pimpinella anisum) 120, 179
Anthraquinones 58
Anti-inflammatory 66, 68, 73, 104, 106
Anti-Nausea 44, 71, 72
Antispasmodic 71, 76, 90
Anxiety 44,56, 66, 68, 90, 106
Ashwagandha (Withania somnifera) 45, 103, 111, 167, 168
Astragalus (Astragalus membranaceus) 45, 65, 103, 173, 179
Astringent 44
Avocado (Persea americana) 103, 145, 146, 158, 160

B

Baobab (Adansonia digitata) 167
Barberry (Berberis vulgaris) 49, 58
Basil (Ocimum basilicum) 57
Bay (Laurus nobilis) 145, 146
Beet Root (Beta vulgaris) 55, 69
Belly Binding 138, 152
Berberine 57, 58
Bitter 72
Black Cohosh (Actaea racemosa) 54, 83, 84, 89,109
Black Walnut (Juglans nigra) 125
Blackhaw (Viburnum prunifolium) 65, 76, 84, 93
Bleeding 44, 85, 90, 92, 111
Blessed Thistle (Cnicus benedictus) 45, 120
Blessing Ceremonies 139
Bloating 44
Blood Pressure 65, 84, 90, 155
Blood Sugar 65, 103
Bloodroot (Sanguinaria canadensis) 58
Blue Cohosh (Caulophyllum thalictroides) 49, 50, 83,89
Blue Vervain (Verbena hastata) 93, 111
Borage (Borago officinalis) 49, 58
Breastfeeding 116-117, 121, 122
Brewer's Yeast (Saccharomyces cerevisiae) 120
Brigid's Well 139
Buckthorn (Rhamnus spp.) 49
Burdock (Arctium lappa) 65, 69, 173,179

C

Cabbage (Brassica oleracea) 126
Cacao (Theobroma cacao) 103, 167, 168
Caffeine 54
Calcium 65, 67, 68, 76, 107
Calendula (Calendula officinalis) 46, 51, 65, 70,111, 112, 125, 145, 146
California Poppy (Eschscholzia califomica) 110
Calmative 44, 66, 68, 106
Camphor (Cinnamomum camphora) 58
Cardamom (Elettaria cardamomum) 57, 179
Cardiovascular 67
Carob (Ceratonia siliqua) 70
Cascara Sagrada (Rhamnus purshiana) 49
Castor Bean (Ricinus communis) 49, 83, 110
Catnip (Nepeta cataria) 109, 123
Celtic Traditions 139
Chamomile (Matricaria chamomilla) 44, 45,56, 57, 65, 70, 75, 112, 125, 146, 158, 179
Chaya (Cnidoscolus aconitifolius) 65
Chickweed (Stellaria media) 65
Chinese Practices 137
Chocolate (Theobroma cacao) 103
Cinnamon (Cinnamomum verum) 57, 65, 76, 103, 123, 145, 146,168, 179
Circulation 67, 69, 77
Clary Sage (Salvia sclarea) 57, 83
Cleavers (Galium aparine) 123, 124
Clove (Syzygium aromaticum) 125
Coconut (Cocos nucifera) 54, 66, 103, 125, 168
Coffee (Coffea arabica or Coffea robusta) 49, 54
Cognitive Function 66, 105
Cold/Cough 66, 73, 75
Coltsfoot (Tussilago farfara) 49, 58
Comfrey (Symphytum officinale) 46, 49, 58, 111, 124, 145, 146
Compress 35
Constipation 57, 68, 69, 107, 155
Contractions 78, 109
Corn Lily (Veratrum spp.) 49
Cornsilk (Zea mays) 44, 69
Cotton Root (Gossypium herbaceum) 49, 52, 83
Coumarins 58
Cradleboard 136
Cramp 50, 65, 71, 76, 90, 92, 103, 104, 109
Crampbark (Viburnum opulus) 71, 76, 93, 104,109,110, 112
Cuarentena 136

D

Damiana (Turnera diffusa) 66, 104 167, 168
Dan Shen (Salvia miltiorrhiza) 104, 179
Dandelion (Taraxacum officinale) 44, 45, 66, 69,71, 76, 104
Dates (Phoenix dactylifera) 86

Decoction 37
Delayed Period 44
Depressants 49, 56
Detoxification 65, 66, 72, 73
Digestive Aids 44, 65, 66, 68, 72, 104
Dill (Anethum graveolens) 86
Diuretic 44, 103
Dong Quai (Angelica sinensis) 54
Druid 139, 140

E

Echinacea (Echinacea purpurea or Echinacea angustifolia) 45, 66, 73, 74, 75, 123, 124
Edema 44, 68, 69, 77
Elderberry (Sambucus nigra) 45, 66, 73, 74
Elderflower (Sambucus nigra) 74
Elecampane (Inula helenium) 66, 73
Electrolytes 66
Eleuthero (Eleutherococcus senticosus) 66, 70, 73, 75
Elixir 35
Emmenagogues 49, 58
Energy 54, 66, 67, 103, 104
Ephedra (Ephedra sinica) 49
Ergot Fungus (Claviceps purpurea) 58
Essential Oils 49
Eucalyptus (Eucalyptus globulus) 75, 158, 160
Evening Primrose Oil (Oenothera biennis) 83

F

Facilitate Labor 77
Fang Fen (Saposhnikovia divaricata) 145
Fatigue 70
Fennel (Foeniculum vulgare) 44, 45, 104, 112
Fenugreek (Trigonella foenum-graecum) 45, 119, 123
Flaxseed (Linum usitatissimum) 57
Focus 66
Frankincense (Boswellia sacra or Boswellia serrata) 57

G

Galactagogues 45, 104, 105, 106, 119, 121
Garlic (Allium sativum) 174
Gas 44
Gestational Diabetes 76
Giant Fennel (Ferula communis) 49
Ginger (Zingiber officinale) 44, 55, 57, 66, 69, 71, 73, 74, 75, 7 6, 104, 109, 123, 145, 146, 164, 179
Gingko (Gingko biloba) 66
Ginseng (Panax ginseng or Panax quinquefolius) 55, 66, 70,109
Global Traditions 136
Goat's Rue (Galega officinalis) 45, 105, 120

Goji Berry (Lycium barbarum) 105, 164
Goldenrod (Solidago spp.) 67
Goldenseal (Hydrastis canadensis) 49, 58
Gotu Kola (Centella asiatica) 105, 110, 123
Grapeseed Extract (Vitis vinifera) 125
Guarana (Paullinia cupana) 49
Guava (Psidium guajava) 105, 158, 160
Guayusa (Ilex guayusa) 54, 55
Guinea Hen (Petiveria alliacea) 145, 146

H

Hawthorne (Crataegus spp) 45, 67, 84, 167, 168
Headache 106
Heart Opener 45, 90, 167, 168
Heartburn 70
Hemlock 49
Hemorrhoid 70
Herbal Actions 43
Herbal Baths 138
Hibiscus (Hibiscus sabdariffa) 167, 179
Holistic Support 24
Holy Basil (Ocimum sanctum) 45, 56, 67, 70, 105, 111, 167
Hops (Humulus lupulus) 49, 58, 67, 105, 112
Hormone Balance 68
Hyssop (Hyssopus officinalis) 58

I

Immunity 45, 65, 67, 68, 73, 103, 105, 107
Indigenous Tradition 136
Infusion 36
Insomnia 56, 70, 112
Insulin Sensitivity 76
Irish Moss, (sea moss, Chondrus crispus) 107
Iron 45, 65, 67, 68, 69, 76, 92, 106

J

Jasmine (Jasminum sambac) 126, 167
Jimsonweed 49
Jujubee (Ziziphus jujuba) 105

K

Kanna (Sceletium tortuosum) 167
Katrafay 44, 105, 145, 146
Kava (Piper methysticum) 49, 56
Kidney 67
Kratom 49, 57

L

Labor 78, 83, 90
Lactation 116-117, 121, 122
Latch 116
Lavender (Lavandula angustifolia) 44, 56, 57, 75, 106, 109, 145, 146, 158, 167
Laxatives 49, 57, 73
Lemon 67, 71, 72
Lemon Balm (Melissa officinalis) 56, 75, 111, 112, 167
Lemongrass 145, 146
Linden (Tilia cordata) 84, 167, 168
Liver 65, 66, 76, 104
Lotus (Nelumbo nucifera) 167
Low plateletes 77
Lucuma 55

M

Maca (Lepidium meyenii) 54, 55, 67, 70
Magnesium 68, 71
Mango 146
Marshmallow Root (Althaea officinalis) 57, 67, 70, 73, 106
Mastitis 123
Matcha 55
Memory 66, 105
MesoAmerican 148
Methyl Salicylate 58
Milk Thistle (Silybum marianum) 120
Miscarriage 76, 92
Mood 45, 56, 66, 67, 68, 90, 92, 103, 104, 105, 111
Moon Rituals 139
Moringa (Moringa oleifera) 67, 106, 123
Morning Sickness 71, 72
Motherwort (Leonurus cardiaca) 45, 51, 90, 93, 109, 110, 111, 123, 167, 168
Moxibustion 137
Mugwort (Artemisia vulgaris) 49, 50, 51, 110, 145, 146, 160
Mullien (Verbascum thapsus) 67, 73, 74, 124
Muscle Cramps 71
Myrhh 145, 146

N

Naming Ceremony 138
Neem 125
Nervine 45
Nettle (Urtica dioica) 44, 45, 67, 69, 70, 71, 76, 93, 106, 109, 110, 112, 126,174
Nightshade 49
Nipple Health 125
Nursing Through 128
Nutmeg (Myristica fragrans) 58
Nutrition 67, 100, 107, 136, 172, 176, 178

O

Oat (Avena sativa) 106, 112, 179
Oats (tops and straw) 45, 123
Oregano 49, 57
Oregon grape (Mahonia aquifolium) 49, 58
Oregon Grape Root 58

P

Papaya (Carica papaya) 46, 106
Parsely 126
Partridge Berry (Mitchella repens) 46, 76, 84, 93, 106
Passionflower (Passiflora incarnata) 49,56, 112
Peach (Prunus persica) 68,71
Pennyroyal (Mentha pulegium) 49, 50, 52, 57
Peppermint 44, 57, 75, 126
Peristeam Hydrotherapy 154
Phytoestrogens 49, 54,
Placenta 136, 162
Placental Abruption 54
Plantain (Musa spp.) 68
Plantain (Plantago major) 46, 73, 86, 107, 146, 158
Poke Root (Phytolacca Decandra) 124
Poppy (Papaver somniferum). 58
Postpartum Baths 144
Postpartum Baths 143
Postpartum Depression 90
Postpartum hemmorrage 86, 90
Postpartum Mood Disorder 45, 90
Postpartum Sitz 111
Poultice 35,39
PPH 86
Pre-eclampsia 77
Psyllium Husk 57, 69

R

Ragwort 49
Rebozo 136
Red Clover (Trifolium pratense) 49, 51, 123
Red Dates 164
Red Raspberry (Rubus idaeus) 44,45,46, 68, 76, 83, 93, 107, 111, 158
Reflection 18
Regulate Menstruation 50
Reishi (Ganoderma lucidum) 45, 167
Respiratory 66, 73
Rhubarb (Rheum rhabarbarum) 49
Ritual 131
Rooibos 54, 55
Rose (Rosa spp.) 45, 68, 107,111, 112, 145, 146, 158, 167,168
Rosehip 74,112
Rosemary(Rosmarinus Officinalis) 57, 145, 146, 158, 160
Rubifacient 75
Rue 49, 50, 52, 145, 146

S

Sacral Steam 154
Safflower 49, 50,
Safrole 58
Sage (Salvia officinalis) 58, 126
Sassafras (Sassafras albidum) 58
Schisandra (Schisandra chinensis) 54, 55, 107,
Scotch Broom 49, 50
Senna (Senna alexandrina) 58
Shatavari (Asparagus racemosus) 119, 123, 167, 168
Shea 145, 146
Shepherd's Purse (Capsella bursa-pastoris) 84, 85, 86, 111
Skin 65, 68, 105, 107, 110
Skullcap (Scutelaria lateriflora) 44, 45, 56, 68, 70, 71, 111, 168
Slippery Elm (Ulmus rubra) 57, 69, 70, 107
Soy (Glycine max) 54
Spearmint (Mentha spicata) 69, 71, 73, 74, 111, 112,123
Spiritual Cleansing 139
Spirulina (Arthrospira platensis (or maxima) 45, 55, 68, 69
Spotting 76
St. Johns Wort 110
Steam 75, 156
Stimulants 49, 54
Stress 66, 67
Sweat Lodge 136
Sweet Birch (Betula lenta) 58
Sweet clover (Melilotus officinalis) 58
Syrup 35,38

T

Tansy (Tanacetum vulgare) 49, 50, 52, 57
Tea Tree 125
Teas 35
Temazcal 136
Teratogens 49, 52, 53
Thrush 125
Thuja 49, 50
Thujone 58
Thyme 57, 173
Tincture 35,40,41
Tobacco 49
Tonic 45
Tonka bean (Dipteryx odorata) 58
Tree Symbolism 140
Turmeric (Curcuma longa) 55, 68, 71, 107, 179

U

Uterine Atony 86
Uterine Tonics 45, 46, 68, 73, 76, 78, 107, 155
Uva Ursi 146

V

Valerian 44, 70
Vitamin K 65, 68, 77
Vitex 111
Vulnerary 46, 107

W

Weaning 122
Wild Yam (Dioscorea villosa) 44, 68,71, 76
Wintergreen (Gaultheria procumbens) 57, 58
Witch Hazel (Hamamelis virginiana) 44, 70, 85,111, 124, 146, 158, 160
Womb Massage 94, 136, 148
Wormwood (Artemisia absinthium) 49, 50, 58, 160
Wu Zhu Yu 145

Y

Yarrow (Achillea millefolium) 44, 46, 49, 50, 51, 85, 93, 124, 126, 145, 146, 158, 167
Yellowdock (Rumex crispus) 45, 57, 68, 69, 107
Yerba Mate 54, 55
Yunnan Baiyo (Proprietary blend including Panax Notoginseng) 85

More From the Rooted Collection

Rooted Online Course:

This informative course is an essential resource for herbalists, birthworkers, midwives, healthcare providers, and expectant mothers seeking holistic support. It will help you navigate the transformative journey of motherhood with confidence, healing, and empowerment.

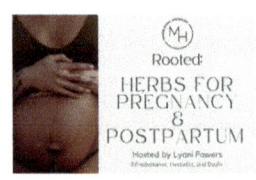

The Rooted: Pregnancy and Postpartum Online Course is a comprehensive and transformative learning experience that blends ancient wisdom with modern practices, providing a holistic approach to maternal wellness. This course covers essential herbs, remedies, and comfort measures that support a healthy pregnancy, postpartum recovery, and lactation journey.

In this course, you'll explore:
- Herbal Support for Pregnancy: Learn which herbs can help support fertility, ease common pregnancy discomforts, and promote optimal health for both mother and baby.
- Postpartum Healing: Discover the power of herbs and natural remedies that aid in physical recovery, emotional well-being, and nourishing the body after childbirth.
- Holistic Approaches: Gain insight into cultural traditions from around the world, and how to integrate these approaches into your care for the maternal dyad.
- Practical Herbal Remedies: Get hands-on with creating and using herbal syrups, poultices, infusions, decoctions, tinctures, and more.
- Materia Medica: Access an extensive guide to herbs that support preconception, pregnancy, lactation, and postpartum care, including safety guidelines and dosage recommendations.

By the end of the course, you'll have the knowledge and tools to provide nurturing, evidence-based care using herbal remedies and ancient traditions, creating a personalized wellness plan for pregnancy, postpartum, and beyond.

Rooted Cookbook:

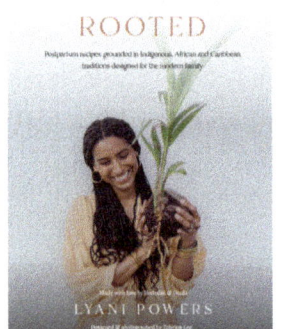

Rooted: Postpartum Recipes Grounded in Indigenous, African, and Caribbean Traditions, Designed for the Modern Family" is a unique cookbook that blends global comfort foods, nourishing new mothers during their golden month and beyond. Celebrating cultural heritage, the book offers a holistic approach to postpartum care, supporting both physical and emotional well-being. More than just recipes, Rooted is a guide to heritage-infused healing for the journey of motherhood.

www.ingramcontent.com/pod-product-compliance
Lightning Source LLC
Chambersburg PA
CBHW052128030426
42337CB00028B/5071